A Doctor remembers

Dr Arthur D. Bethune, MB ChB

Arth D. Beth

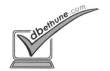

first published in 2013 by dbethune.com, Selkirk, Scotland

text © Arthur D. Bethune, 2012
layout © David R. Bethune, 2013

Arthur D. Bethune has asserted his right under the Copyright,
Designs and Patents Act 1988 to be identified as the author of
this work

All rights reserved.
No part of this publication may be reproduced, stored in a
retrieval system or transmitted in any form or by any means
electronic, mechanical, photocopying, recording or otherwise,
without the prior written permission of the publishers and
copyright owner.

Printed and bound in Belfast by W&G Baird

ISBN 978-0-9576779-0-6

All proceeds from the sale of this book will go to support
Newcastleton Community First Responders
Scottish Charity No SC037944
http://www.visitnewcastleton.com/content/first-responders

further copies available from 01750 21703

cover picture: view up Liddesdale from Penton

THE ROYAL INFIRMARY.

□ □ □

This is to certify that *Arthur B. Bethune*

has this day taken out a Perpetual Ticket for the Medical Surgical Practice of this Hospital.

Henry Shaw.

Treasurer.

EDINBURGH, *16th April* 194 *2*

This Ticket, which is issued subject to the Regulations of the Managers, entitles the Holder to visit the Wards and Operating Theatres, and attend Post-Mortem Examinations.

It must be shown at the Treasurer's office once every month when Cards are called, for the purpose of recording Hospital Attendance; and no Certificate of regular attendance can be given to any Student who does not comply with this Regulation.

No. 410

The author's student pass for the Royal Infirmary, Edinburgh, issued 16th April 1942

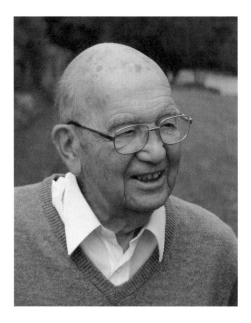

These "rememberings" were first printed as a series of articles in the Copshaw Clatter between 2009 and 2012. Initially, there were to be just a few, but once started, the stories just kept on coming and coming.

Eventually, after 32 monthly columns, the series came to a natural end point, and so my family decided to bring them together, with some old photographs, maps and illustrations, in this small book.

The book is dedicated to the Newcastleton Community First Responders, who do so much of the "out of hours" work that we old doctors used to do, and to the superb team of Social Work carers in Newcastleton to whom I owe so much.

I hope you enjoy reading these "memoirs".

Arthur Bethune, Newcastleton, 2013

Contents

Acknowledgements

The publishers would like to thank the following for their kind permission

(a) to reproduce their photographs:

Arthur Bethune: iii, vi, 2, 5, 8, 11, 14, 15, 16, 22, 26, 44, 47, 48, 49, 51, 61, 64(ii), 71, 75, 76(i), 82, 86, 90, 94(i), 95(i,ii)
David Bethune: cover, 25, 34, 38, 42, 52, 62, 66, 70, 76(i), 78(both), 79, 80(ii), 87, 88, 89, 92, 94(ii), 96
Oliver Dixon: 45 (from www.geograph.co.uk, licenced for use under Creative Commons Licence)
Walter Baxter: 55 (licenced for use under Creative Commons Licence
Bill Lynn: 56, 57
the Marshall family: 64(i)
the Cuthbert family: 65
Cecilia Davidson: 72
public domain, Wikimedia Commons: 1, 3, 43, 69, 80(i), 83, 85
public domain, Scotland from the roadside gallery: 24
Ships Nostalgia collection: 54

(b) to use their drawings, sketches and maps:

Andrew Bethune: 7, 10(map), 13, 23, 35, 47, 53, 67, 84
Arthur Bethune: 12
Frances Bethune: 29
Mary Vander Steen: 37
David Bethune: 41, 46, 93
Nick Bethune: 59, 63
Louise Raffier: 71, 72, 74, 77, 81
freeworldmaps.net, adapted: 30

(c) to scan and print documents:

Matthew Shaw of timetableworld.com: timetable on page 10
Arthur Bethune: hospital pass on page ii, tickets and rail passes on pages 10, 57, 58 and old postcards on pages 18 and 20

Thanks are also due to the editorial team of the **Copshaw Clatter** for permission to re-use the text originally printed as monthly articles between 2009 and 2012.

Every effort has been made to trace the copyright holders and we apologise in advance for any unintentional omissions or inaccuracies. We would be pleased to insert the appropriate acknowledgement in any subsequent edition of this publication.

Introduction

Canty Bay is a lovely sandy bay a few miles east of North Berwick, opposite the Bass Rock. The old fishermen's cottages there were given to the Scouts through the generosity of W. Edgar Evans, a scientist at the Edinburgh Royal Botanical Gardens and a former Scoutmaster.

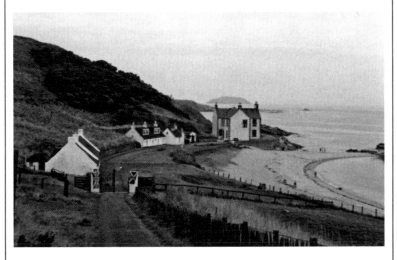

It was there on 19th April 1936, when I was 12, and in one of these bare walled cottages that, at a Scout Scripture Union meeting, "Pa Evans" as we affectionately called him, helped me understand for the first time in my life the basic truths of the Christian faith – Jesus' death on the cross for our sins, the need for repentance and faith in Him. It was the start of my slow journey to a personal faith in Jesus which dominated my life and the way I practised medicine.

Arthur Bethune, 2013

1. Medicine without Paracetamol

Returning from hospital recently with a batch of drugs, most of which were new to me, I started to think about what drugs were available when I was a medical student during the war.

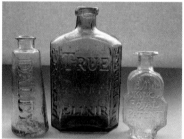

For relief of pain we only had aspirin, phenacetin (from which paracetamol was later derived), caffeine and codeine, apart from the strong opiates like morphia. Caffeine is not used now but a related drug, theophylline, is still used as a bronchodilator.

One day in 1944, the surgical registrar in Mr Paterson-Brown's ward in Edinburgh Royal Infirmary told us that he had just received a letter from a friend in the army with news of a new drug called penicillin, which was doing wonders. However it would be a couple of years before it was freely available. The only antibiotics were the sulphonamides, the most famous being sulphapyridine

M&B 693, which at this time was a great advance in the treatment of pneumonia.

The other potent drugs were liver injections for pernicious anaemia (now superseded by Vitamin B12) and the early simple insulins for diabetes. We had phenobarbitone and barbiturate sleeping tablets, digoxin and painful injections called mersalyl for heart failure, and glyceryl trinitrate tablets to put under your tongue for angina. For asthma there were only ephedrine tablets and adrenaline injections, and a related drug ergometrine to control bleeding after childbirth.

Research about cortisone was in progress, and to treat Addison's Disease we had an unreliable steroid implant called D.O.C.A.

APT injections were available to immunise children against diphtheria. (Actually, I have seen only one case of diphtheria in my career). And there was, of course, smallpox vaccination.

Before the advent of the NHS in 1948, the poor of Edinburgh city centre (the Royal Mile etc) received free medical care from the Cowgate dispensary ('The Cowgate' it was called) run by the Edinburgh Medical Missionary Society. There was a resident doctor but we, as senior students, did the housecalls and called in the resident doctors if the case was serious.

I went visiting with fellow student, Leslie Stokoe, who later became an eye specialist in Edinburgh, and recall visiting a child with congenital heart disease on the top floor (4th, I think) in a tall tenement at the top of The Mound. That child would never be able to go out but he had a fantastic view over the Firth of Forth to Fife.

2. Penicillin at last

The word scurvy conjures up pictures of sailors on sailing ships on long sea voyages in the past, but, when I was a student in Edinburgh, old men from the lodging houses in the city centre came to the Infirmary Outpatients Dept. with scurvy. This was because they lived on soup (in which all the vitamin C had been destroyed) and bread. On one occasion, when the nurse pulled off an old man's socks, the dust billowed into the air. I suspect they had not been off for months!

After graduation, my first job was as a House Physician at Edinburgh Western General Hospital.

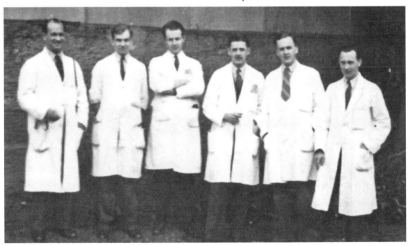

A young-looking Dr. Bethune (2nd from left) with colleagues at the Western General in 1945

2

There were only five resident doctors plus three Polish doctors at the nearby Paderewski Hospital and Polish Medical School, housed as a wartime emergency in a former children's home.

The Western General was run by a Medical Superintendent and by a Matron who was in charge of nursing and cleaning.

My boss was Dr J. G. Sclater. He was interested in rheumatology and six beds in my wards were set aside for patients with rheumatoid arthritis etc.

This was before the steroid era, and gold injections were the mainstay of treatment. This could damage the blood cells and patients were required to have a blood count before each weekly injection. We didn't have technicians to take the blood and we had to do the blood counts ourselves in the ward lab. We also made plaster of Paris removable splints for the patients' hands to ease arthritis pain. Dr Sclater had a rheumatic clinic at the Royal Infirmary and I went up to help him (travelling by bus of course). I think this would be the start of the Rheumatology clinic in Edinburgh.

This was my first chance to handle penicillin. It was so scarce we had to have special permission to use it and this happened only twice in my six months there. Penicillin came as hard tablets and it was my job to prepare it for use by shaking it up in a litre of cold water.

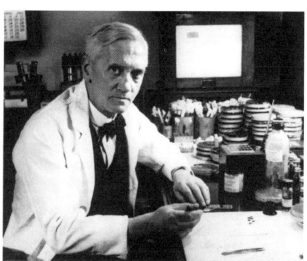

Sir Alexander Fleming, discoverer of penicillin

Strangely enough, my son, David, married a relative; his wife's great-great-grandfather was Sir Alexander Fleming's uncle!

This took half an hour and the penicillin was ready to be run into a patient's thigh muscle all day by drip.

It was wartime and many consultants were away in the army, so those left behind were busy. That's why, at the age of 21, I was left with a lot of responsibility, as Dr Sclater did not normally visit my wards on Saturday, Sunday and Monday.

There were lighter moments. One confused patient in my ward complained about "the nasty woman who keeps the picture house." We puzzled over this and then realised it was the night nurse who came after the lights were out - with a torch, like an usherette in the cinema.

She wasn't 'nasty' - I took her out quite a number of times!

3. Into General Practice

"If you are going to be a GP you will have to wear a hat" – so said my sister.

So I went to Aitken & Niven's menswear shop where my friend, Jack Cochrane, sold me a suitable hat for 7/6. (37½p). The war was nearly over and the Government decided to send us newly qualified doctors for 6 months to help the tired, elderly GPs before sending us to the army. Actually I never got into the army as I was medically unfit.

In those days a GP needed to be properly dressed – not only a hat, but a dark suit with a waistcoat and a white shirt and tie.

To add to the professional image, my first boss, Dr George Sinclair of Lockerbie, kept a pair of white gloves in the car, which he picked up and carried into the patient's house. He never wore them.

On my arrival at Lockerbie station, Dr Sinclair said, "Do you usually wear a hat?" I said, "No", and never wore the hat again! My Uncle Nichol fell heir to it some years later.

Five years later, I had difficulty persuading the late Dr Jimmy Murdoch that it was not unprofessional to drive about the practice with your jacket off on a boiling hot day.

4

The flags were out for my arrival in Lockerbie, and the next day was declared a public holiday, though that may have had something to do with the end of the war! It was 16th August 1945.

Life in a rural area was all new to me. Dr Sinclair took me around for a few days and then let me loose on a trusting public. It was very scary being shut into the surgery on your own. Worse was to come. Within 10 days, Dr Sinclair left me alone and went off to Lairg for a few days to buy North Country Cheviot lambs, which he sold on to his farmer patients. His father had been a herd in Caithness. There was a home confinement at Dryfe Bridge while he was away but all went well.

One problem which I had before coming to Lockerbie was that I had only driven a car three times on the road! Driving tests were in abeyance during the war. One of the earliest things I did was to drive to Eskdalemuir in the dark to calm a farmer who had celebrated too much after the sales…

On the way up, I saw the lights of a big village ahead, which surprised me. The lights turned out to be light reflected from the eyes of a flock of sheep resting on the tarmac road.

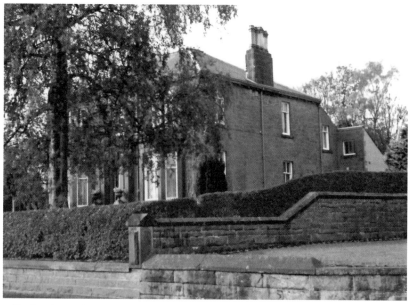

Dr Sinclair's house and surgery in Lockerbie, taken on a return visit in 1993

4. More from Lockerbie

I did three surgeries a day, six days a week, and was on call all the time apart from a weekend off once a month. I would catch the 8.30 pm train to Edinburgh after doing the Friday night surgery and had to be back on the Monday in time for the evening surgery at 7 pm, as the doctor always went to play bridge on Monday nights.

Looking back, I think we juniors were exploited by the senior doctors, but we were young, unmarried and accepted full-time work as the norm and the only way to gain experience.

In 1945, the NHS was still almost three years away and so we had two kinds of patients – 'panel' and 'private'. The so-called 'panel' patients were those covered by the Lloyd George Insurance scheme for employed persons. These were entitled to a free doctor and to medicines, but the rest (wives, children and self-employed) had to pay for everything.

There were two chemists in Lockerbie. The 'panel' patients got all their medicines from them. The private patients got some bottles of medicine and ointments from the doctor, so I had to learn how to dispense. We had a 'nerve tonic' containing phenobarbitone and a 'pick-me-up' strychnine tonic. One patient said to me "That tonic gave me a real kick!' No wonder! She had been taking a tablespoonful instead of the labelled teaspoonful of the strychnine tonic. Four times the dose! When asked if she had read the label she said that she hadn't but that the last time she had some medicine it had said a tablespoonful.

After the bottles were mixed, they were corked and neatly labelled. There were sheets of white paper in which they were carefully wrapped. Then they were sealed with sealing wax. (We were still using sealing wax even in my early days in Newcastleton).

Few records were kept, mainly those of the visits done and the medicines dispensed. These were essential for subsequent charging. Dr Sinclair said, "If you start writing things down, your memory goes".

What a difference from the mass of paperwork today!

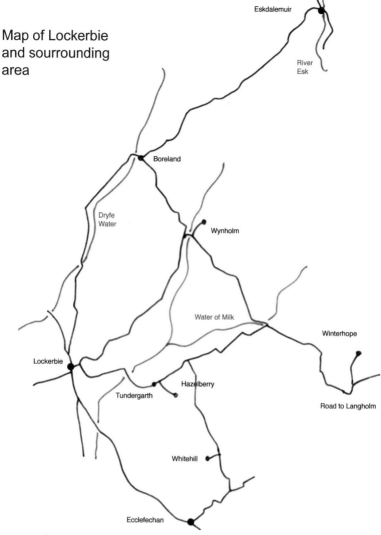

Map of Lockerbie and sourrounding area

Eskdalemuir

River
Esk

Boreland

Dryfe
Water

Wynholm

Water of Milk

Winterhope

Lockerbie

Hazelberry

Tundergarth

Road to Langholm

Whitehill

Ecclefechan

In many Scottish rural practices, the rich subsidised the poor and Lockerbie was no exception. I recall going to a cottage on the Annan road and then on some 100 yards to a big country house. The cottager was charged 7/6, the lady in the big house £1.1.0.

Following a confinement, the last of the postnatal visits involved vaccinating the baby against smallpox. This was compulsory unless you signed a document to say you did not believe in it. Smallpox was not then a disease of the past.

There was an outbreak of it in Edinburgh Royal Infirmary when I was a student and also a number of cases in Glasgow.

There were farm accidents. I attended a man tossed by a bull at Wynholm, and another attacked by a cow in the Mart.

Tyres were very scarce and we had to run them till they were threadbare. Punctures were a frequent occurrence. Once I had to change a wheel in the dark near Boreland by the light of an auriscope (the instrument for examining the ear). Eventually, after two punctures in a day,

I got a permit for two new tyres, but that wasn't the end of the story. The garage had not secured the wheels properly and one broke on the rough road to Winterhope (between Lockerbie and Langholm).

On another occasion, the track rod fell off one wheel and I had to get out and kick the wheel round at sharp bends.

Although I had been used to camping in the country, it was a surprise to find houses off the road such as Hazelberry, a mile up from Tundergarth Farm, and the Upper Whitehill Cottage (where the uncle of the late Mrs Currie of Newlands lived), across a field, through a gate, across another field and through a fence. I am sure there must have been a better way to it from the Ecclefechan side!

(Tundergarth was where the nose section of Pan Am flight 103 crashed to earth some 40 years later)

This was good preparation for my next job where many houses were much further off the road. There were more adventures with ageing cars to come!

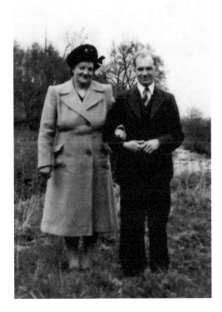

with my landlady, Mrs. Irving, in Lockerbie, 1949

5. Off to the Hebrides

Tuesday 26th February 1946 saw me heading for Kyle of Lochalsh on the evening train from Inverness. It was a snowy night. There were two other passengers in the compartment and they conversed in Gaelic with never a word to me in English. Dr Macleod of Lochmaddy in North Uist had written to ask me to come there as his assistant when I finished my six months in Lockerbie.

I had been recommended by Chrissie Matheson, the head midwife in Edinburgh who was a friend of the Macleods. She had been a patient of mine in the Western General Hospital. Somehow I managed to persuade the War Committee to let me go, and so here I was off to catch the 550-ton steamer 'Lochmor' at Kyle. I was the only non-Gaelic speaker on board. (It was not the tourist season and visitors to the Uists were few and far between then, six months after the war). Fortunately, I shared a 2-berth cabin with a young army officer from Harris who showed me the ropes. However he said, "Uist? It's a wild place!" I wondered what I had let myself in for!

I woke the next morning to find the 'Lochmor' off the northwest coast of Skye, and, after stops at Scalpay Island, Tarbert in Harris, and two small places on the coast of Harris where small boats came out to meet the steamer, got to Lochmaddy at 5.30 pm – 32 hours after leaving Edinburgh – and was met by Dr Macleod. He was dressed, not in the Lockerbie style, but with a thick pullover with a roll-top neck. The next day he told me I was too well dressed and sent me back to get older clothing on! A travel writer wrote he was 'more like a Battersea bruiser than a doctor.'

Lochmaddy, on the east coast of the island, is the administrative centre, but most people lived on the fertile west side 7 to 15 miles away.

The next morning, we set off for the west in the doctor's old Ford car – YS something (the rest of the number plate was missing!) The passenger seat was also missing so I sat in the back, blissfully unaware that the road went along a raised causeway (with no barrier) over Loch Scadavaig, and that the doctor had only one eye, as he peered

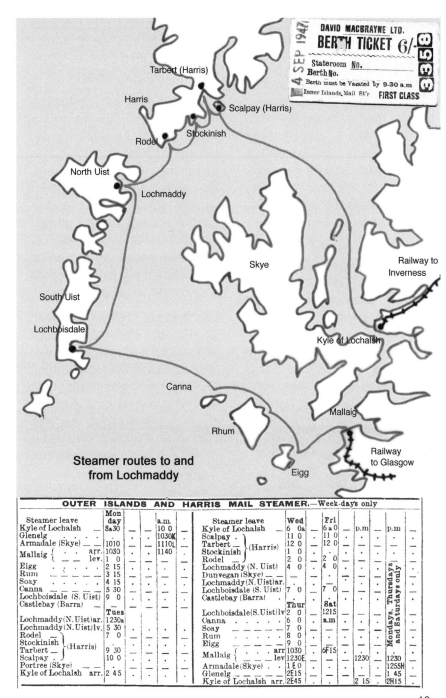

Tarbert (Harris)

Harris

Scalpay (Harris)

Stockinish

Rodel

North Uist

Lochmaddy

Skye

Railway to Inverness

South Uist

Lochboisdale

Kyle of Lochalsh

Canna

Mallaig

Rhum

Railway to Glasgow

Eigg

Steamer routes to and from Lochmaddy

DAVID MACBRAYNE LTD.
BERTH TICKET 6/-
4 SEP 1947
3358
Stateroom No.
Berth No.
Berth must be Vacated by 9-30 a.m
Inner Islands Mail St'r   FIRST CLASS

OUTER ISLANDS AND HARRIS MAIL STEAMER.—Week-days only				
Steamer leave	Monday		a.m.	
Kyle of Lochalsh	8a30	—	10 0	.
Glenelg	.	.	1030K	.
Armadale (Skye)	1010	.	1110L	.
Mallaig { arr.	1030	.	1140	.
{ lev.	1 0	.	.	.
Eigg	2 15	.	.	.
Rum	3 15	—	.	—
Soay	4 15	.	.	.
Canna	5 30	.	.	—
Lochboisdale (S. Uist)	9 0	.	.	.
Castlebay (Barra)	—			
	Tues			
Lochmaddy(N.Uist)ar.	1230a	.	.	.
Lochmaddy(N.Uist)lv.	5 30	.	.	—
Rodel	7 0	.	.	—
Stockinish }(Harris)				
Tarbert }	9 30	.	.	—
Scalpay .	10 0	.	.	—
Portree (Skye)	—	—	.	.
Kyle of Lochalsh arr.	2 45	.	.	.

Steamer leave	Wed	Fri	p.m	p.m	
Kyle of Lochalsh	6 0a	6a0	.	.	
Scalpay .	11 0	11 0	.	.	
Tarbert } (Harris)	12 0	12 0	.	.	
Stockinish }	1 0	.	.	.	
Rodel	2 0	2 0	.	.	
Lochmaddy (N. Uist)	4 0	4 0	.	.	
Dunvegan (Skye)	.	.	.	.	
Lochmaddy(N.Uist)ar.	.	.	.	.	
Lochboisdale (S. Uist)	7 0	7 0	.	.	
Castlebay (Barra)	.	.	.	.	
	Thur	Sat			Mondays, Thursdays and Saturdays only
Lochboisdale(S.Uist)lv	2 0	1215	.	.	
Canna	6 0	a.m	.	.	
Soay	7 0	.	.	.	
Rum	8 0	.	.	.	
Eigg	9 0	.	.	.	
Mallaig { arr	1030	6F15	.	.	
{ lev	1230E	—	1230	1230	
Armadale(Skye)	1 E 0	.	.	1255H	
Glenelg	2E15	.	.	1 45	
Kyle of Lochalsh arr.	2E45	.	2 15	2H15	

10

through the snowy windscreen making the wipers go manually with one arm out the window!

In addition to the 'mainland' of North Uist, the practice covered three other islands, Grimsay and Baleshare (which were tidal) and Berneray. There was a 3-bedded hospice for maternity cases, etc. We had an X-ray machine but insufficient electric power to use it!

We had surgeries at Lochmaddy on Wednesday or Friday afternoons, the days the steamer came in, a surgery on Tuesdays in the Nurse's home at Carinish at the south end, and on Thursday afternoon we saw patients at the crossroads at Bayhead on the west side! Here, we saw a few patients at the roadside (or in the Post Office if it was wet). Nurse Macdonald then took us to see other patients in the area.

Grimsay was two miles by boat, but if the tide was out it was three miles walking and a further three miles to Kallin at the far end of the island. Baleshare was closer, and I usually walked there, though I once went in a horse and cart with the postman. On my first visit to Berneray, we embarked on a small dinghy off the rocks and transferred to a motorboat.

Lochportain, on the far side of Loch Maddy, was three miles by sea and then a two mile walk to the small community of Hoebeg. My first crossing to Lochportain was on a very stormy day with waves lashing into the boat. I lay under a tarpaulin all the way.

Many houses were well off the road, but all have roads now and the three islands have causeways.

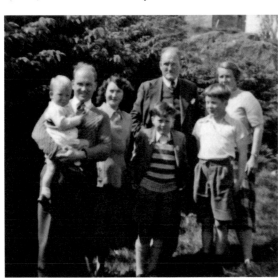

with Dr Macleod and his family in Lochmaddy, on a return visit there in 1952

6. Come at once

On Berneray, a small island off the north end of North Uist, I was faced with a child with severe abdominal pain for which there was no obvious cause. Going back an hour or two later was not an option as it had already taken over an hour to get there. Hospitalisation would mean a small boat journey and an air ambulance. An old, experienced nurse suggests to this young inexperienced doctor, "Why not try an enema?" The result produced at least a pound of currants and an immediate cure! The boy had spent the previous day in his uncle's shop and had stuffed himself with them.

A man came to me one evening. "I think I have broken my wrist starting the lorry." He had indeed! The broken bones were sticking out through the skin. He went off by air ambulance to Glasgow the next morning. That was the only time I used the air ambulance but I did send a Grimsay man to Glasgow by the regular air service from Benbecula. The plane was a small Rapide. The man had bladder problems so we sat him in the back seat with a bottle in case of emergency.

There was one occasion when moving an extremely ill patient was not an option. She lived two miles away by sea, and then a further two miles by footpath. This 17-year old girl was unconscious with neck rigidity. In fact, she had meningitis. At that time, we were one of the few practices with a small stock of penicillin because of our remoteness. I started 4-hourly injections of penicillin and sulphapyridine at 1.10 pm and continued until 7 am the next morning. By then she was part-conscious. I returned to base and the district nurse went out and continued injections for another three days. She was still alive 15 years ago.

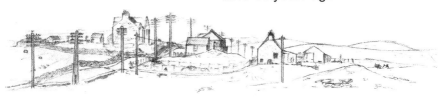

This is a sketch I made at the time of the view from my "digs" at Temple View, Carinish, North Uist.

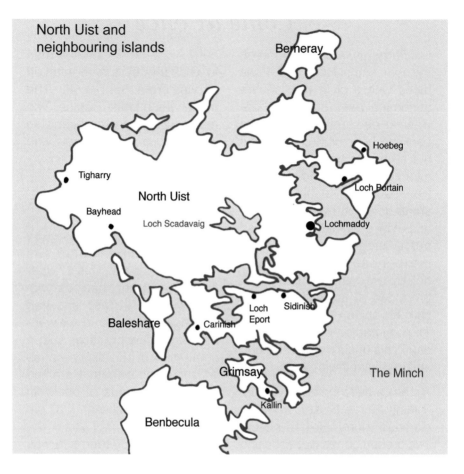

North Uist and neighbouring islands

Berneray

Hoebeg

Tigharry

North Uist

Loch Portain

Bayhead

Loch Scadavaig

Lochmaddy

Loch Eport

Sidinish

Baleshare

Carinish

Grimsay

The Minch

Kallin

Benbecula

My boss sent me to stay at Carinish at the south end of the island for two months. One day, after driving over a very bumpy road, the rear end of the Ford car (see previous chapter) collapsed onto the road. Neil Chisholm, the mechanic, uncle of Mr Chisholm the dentist who used to come to Newcastleton, discovered that the chassis had broken in two places - it had only been held up by the brake cable! This explained why the brake had been slipping off for some weeks. The result was I was car-less and had to do a lot of extra walking and sometimes travelling by bicycle or by bus or even getting lifts on lorries.

One mode of transport new to me was by horse. One late evening, a man arrived by horse with an extra horse for me, to fetch me to come and see his mother who had a nose bleed. I had never ridden before but somehow I just jumped on and we set off for three miles along the sands to his home – an old house with the fire in the centre and a hole in the corner of the roof to let the smoke out! By the time we got there, the bleeding had stopped. It was now dark and the tide had come in so we had to ride back to Carinish over the moor. I have not been on a horse since then (64 years ago)!

There were no private telephones at that time, only lines between the post offices, so we often received messages by telegram. At 11 am one morning I got one.

'Come at once – Mary Macleod'. (not her real name)

It was a stormy day and, when I asked Hector at Carinish Inn to take me over to Grimsay in his horse and trap (see below), he said he could not as the tide would not go out sufficiently because of the weather. So I arranged with Ewan Nicholson, the Grimsay ferryman, to collect me in the afternoon when he came across for the mailbags.

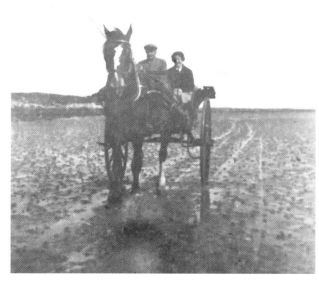

Hector crossing the "North Ford" between North Uist and Grimsay at low tide, with Nurse Fraser, 1946

Because of the weather he had to land ½ mile from Carinish P.O. and we had to carry the mailbags there. We left at 5pm and because it was rough, it took an hour for the two mile crossing to Grimsay. (I may add we had no life belts, life jackets, oars or distress flares.)

After reaching Grimsay, I had an hour's walk to the patient and discovered it was Mary Macleod (Senior), who had shingles. Mary Macleod (Junior) was expecting a baby, but it was not due. I walked back to Grimsay P.O. and stayed there until 10pm when the tide went out enough for me to do the hour's walk back home. The post office was a good place to wait as Mrs Nicholson was a good baker. She had been born in the remote Monach Islands and she lived till she was over 100.

When Mary Macleod Jnr *did* go into labour, Hector took the district nurse and myself in his trap over the tide crack and left us to walk a mile with all our equipment. All went well and we went back by the husband's boat in the early morning.

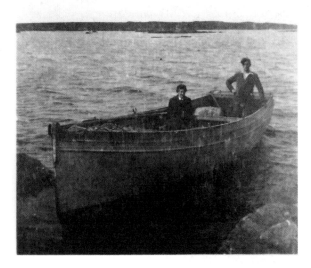

Ewan Nicholson and Nurse Fraser on the Grimsay "ferry", 1946

On the next page, there is another photo of the "ferry" with Joyce on board on our return visit to North Uist in 1952, 6 years later.

7. Nearly a disaster

Colin Macdonald was another assistant of Dr Macleod of Lochmaddy. He always wore a deer-stalker hat. His father, Colin 'Mor', was a member of the Crofting Commission and wrote several amusing books about crofting life.

One night, we nearly had a disaster. We were at a confinement on the west side of the island. The labour was not going well and some help was needed. Horror of horrors! We opened the maternity bag – the forceps were there, but the chloroform was missing. I had to drive full speed the eight miles to Lochmaddy to get some. It was a misty night, the car lights were poor and the brakes did not work, and the route included the curved unprotected causeway over Loch Scadavaig. Because of the delay, the baby was almost dead. Chrissie Matheson, the midwife friend of the Macleods, was on holiday on the island and she 'specialled' the baby for three days. Years later, I walked over some Skye hills with the 'baby' now a fit young boy, while my daughter Frances, aged two, was picking up Gaelic words from his young sister, also two.

There was a measles epidemic. A boy from Tigharry, who had been sent to Glasgow with appendicitis, developed measles shortly after his return home. It was interesting to trace all the contacts as the disease spread from school to school and into the adult population along the west coast. One elderly lady of 80 was a victim, but she made a good recovery.

One morning, I walked out 2½ miles to see a patient. As soon as I got back home to Carinish, a man from Grimsay arrived with a boat to take me to see his ill son at Lameric cottage. However, he was unable to bring me back again as the tide had gone out and landed me half a mile beyond the house I had just visited. Eight miles walk and only two patients seen!

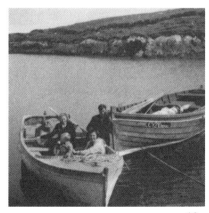

8. From Lochmaddy to Dumfries

The dentist, Richard A Luth, came to Lochmaddy only once every three months, so it fell to the doctor to do any emergency dental treatment. Dr Colin developed severe toothache, so Dr Macleod's help was needed. He gave Colin a whiff of anaesthetic and the pair ran round the surgery twice until Dr Macleod pulled the offending tooth out!

This reminds me that when I first came to Newcastleton, a patient came one Saturday night with severe toothache for me to extract the tooth. I knew the theory and I had Dr Evans' bag of dental forceps but I had never actually taken a tooth out. Not willing to admit this, I tried to put him off by saying, "I am not very good at this." However, he was prepared to take the risk and, amazingly, the molar tooth came out intact! That was the only tooth I have ever extracted.

In 1946, there was a Post Office rule that, if there was an infectious disease in the postman's home, the postman had to stay at home on sick care.

The Grimsay postman's child had whooping cough, so he stayed off on paid sick leave. His son went on as relief postman! Apparently the rule did not apply to temporary postmen!

We had an old man who needed frequent catheterisation. He could have gone to Glasgow for operative treatment but, understandably, Murdo was unwilling to go. The trouble was that he lived two miles off the road, so we trained a neighbour to do the catheterisation and he did so as needed. This had an unexpected complication. I needed a catheter for someone in the middle of the night so I had to go the ten miles to Lochmaddy to get one.

1946 was before the National Health Service and there was a special provision for the remote and sparsely populated areas of the Highlands and Island where medical practice was not financially viable. It was called the Highlands and Islands Medical Service. The doctor was salaried and a house and surgery were provided by the local authority. In addition to his salary, the doctor was allowed to charge a small fee per visit: 1/- (5p).

During my time in Uist I took the long journey to London – 12 hours by boat, followed by 25 hours in the train from Kyle of Lochalsh – and was accepted by the Baptist Missionary Society to go to North China to work at Tai-yuan in Shanxi province.

I arrived back in Uist exactly a week later. The B.M.S. decided that I should get some surgical experience first, so on the evening of 31st August I arrived at Dumfries and Galloway Infirmary to be a house surgeon for a year. As soon as I arrived, I had to stitch a cut in the Outpatient Department, and then a boy arrived with a supracondylar fracture of his arm (a serious injury), so it was very late before I arrived at my ward S3M (Surgical 3 Male).

The night nurse had all the patients settled and was sitting at her desk. Her name was Joyce White! I never dreamed that she would be my future wife!

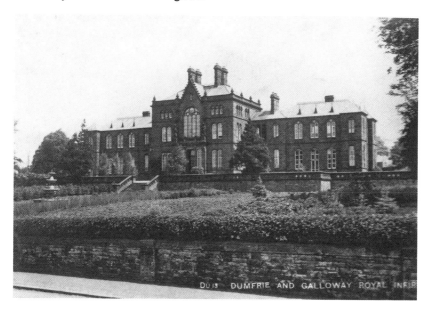

Dumfries Royal Infirmary (from an old postcard)

9. Back to Hospital

As its name implies, Dumfries and Galloway Royal Infirmary, though only a small hospital of about 300 beds, served the needs of the three counties: Dumfriesshire, the Stewartry of Kirkcudbright and Wigtownshire. This was pre-NHS so it was a 'voluntary' hospital, which meant it was financed by legacies, donations and fund-raising. There were two surgical units, one ward under Dr Gordon Hunter and the second a unit of two beds under Mr R. L. Beveridge. The difference was that the latter unit took all the orthopaedic and fracture cases.

Mr Beveridge, my boss, known affectionately as 'Bev', was a perfect gentleman and an excellent surgeon. He had started in Dumfries as a GP surgeon but was now a full-time surgeon. He had an assistant, John Neilson, and a surgical registrar, Jimmy Jack, who was later to become orthopaedic surgeon at Blackburn in Lancashire.

Gordon Hunter was a GP surgeon and unpredictable. Sometimes he would come in to do his ward round after the nurses had the patients settled for the night, and have all the lights turned on again. He had been known to ring up to say he was unable to do his surgical list in the forenoon (after the patients were prepared) and would do it in the evening. I never liked giving an anaesthetic for him. He was too impatient.

The other wards were medical (under Dr Laurie), gynaecology (Dr Bruce Dewar), combined ENT (ears, nose and throat) and eyes, and the children's ward (a mixture of medical and surgical).

There were visiting consultants from Carlisle – Mr Venters (ENT), Dr Leslie Fraser (eyes), and from Glasgow – Mr T. Millar (orthopaedics).

The rest of the medical staff lived in, in a separate house across the road from the Infirmary – the medical registrar and three house surgeons (of which I was one). The house physician lived at the Grove Convalescent Home, out in the country,

We were a happy crowd. No one drank heavily and often in the late evening we sang, round the piano, old songs like Bonnie Galloway and the Lost Chord, sometimes to the annoyance of the Sisters who lived in another detached house next door. One Sister rang up at 2 am to ask when the noise would stop.

Most of the nurses were in their 4-year training and lived in the hospital. It was rare for a ward sister or staff nurse to be married. And, of course, there was a matron, Miss Hutt, who saw that the wards were run efficiently and kept clean.

Of our group, Ian Wilson (who had been an R.A.M.C. doctor on the Normandy beaches on D-Day) became the consultant physician at Kilmarnock Infirmary, John Gibson became anaesthetist at Ashington,

Isabel Kingan became ENT consultant at Dumfries, and Hector McLean became GP on the Small Isles.

As house surgeons, we had no set hours. We just worked all day as needed and got out if things were quiet and one of our colleagues would stand in for us. We had a half-day once a week (but it might not start until mid-afternoon if busy), and a weekend off once a month. We assisted at operations and gave most of the anaesthetics.

The hospital anaesthetist (Charlie Stewart) was a GP and came in only for special cases.

We had no ward secretaries.

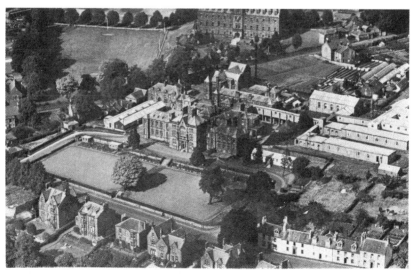

Aeriel view of Dumfries Royal Infirmary, with the staff houses in the foreground

10. More from Dumfries

On my first weekend in Dumfries, a football player was brought in with a serious injury. His name was Jackie Law but, having been brought up in a rugby world, I was unaware that he was a top Queen of the South player, nor had I ever heard of Palmerston Park!

There were no outpatient appointments. Doctors sent patients in with a letter on the advertised outpatients' day. We seemed to manage to see everybody without difficulty. One patient arrived with his doctor's visiting card inscribed on the back, "?Hernia. ?What."

Mr Beveridge, with his sense of humour wrote back, "Hernia. W.L." (waiting list)

Returning to hospital work after a year in North Uist, I found that penicillin was now freely available, though we still had to work out the correct dosage.

In 2010, when I was a patient in the Cardiology Dept. at Carlisle, I was amazed at the number and sophistication of the ECG machines. When I went to Dumfries, there was only **one** ECG machine and it did not work very well.

Hospitals use masses of blood now. At Dumfries in 1946, we only had six bottles of blood in store. Two bottles came from Glasgow once a week. If they were unused we returned them three weeks later, as the shelf life of blood is four weeks.

Once, after a hysterectomy, a patient of mine developed gas gangrene, a serious infection when gas develops under the skin. Part of the treatment was to give a transfusion of fresh blood. I had to take the blood from a relative using make-shift equipment in the hospital lab. I am glad to say she recovered (that is, the patient, as well as the relative).

Radium also came from Glasgow to treat patients with cervical cancer. We had it for a week and treated a number of cases. It was my job as gynaecology house surgeon to insert the radium.

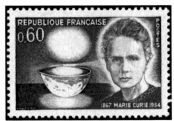

Marie Curie - who discovered Radium and its medical use

One day, the relative peace of the hospital was shattered by a high-pitched regular whistle. It came from a young boy who had inhaled a small spiral shell at the seaside.

It had become stuck in his larynx and he whistled each time he breathed in or out. Fortunately Bob Venters (ENT surgeon) was in Dumfries that day and he got it out.

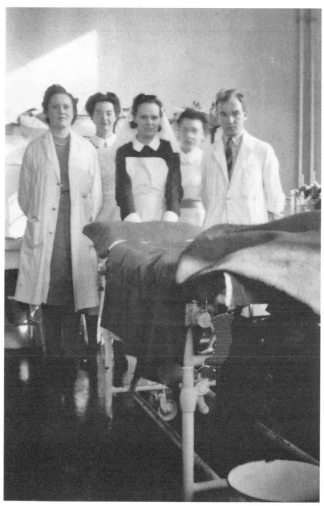

In the operating theatre, Dumfries Royal Infirmary, 1946

We removed a lot of healthy appendices. A burst appendix was a very serious thing in those days with quite a high mortality without antibiotics and a proper understanding of intravenous drips. If there was any doubt, out came the appendix! One day, when Mr Beveridge was repairing a boy's hernia, the appendix popped out of the hernia sac and was removed. (see p.37).

One evening, I gave the anaesthetic to a lady whose appendix was on the point of bursting. I had had symptoms of appendicitis all day and reported sick after the operation. The result was that I landed on the operating table myself!

Another day, a Dumfries doctor sent in a patient with "acute appendicitis". She was actually in full labour, so we passed her on to Cresswell Hospital where she was delivered.

Another job, not strictly my remit, was in the Children's Ward. Nurse May Macmillan made me help her to bottle feed a baby.

In the Children's Ward, the night nurse made the night nurses' supper. I rescued it one night as the nurse was about to put the chips into cold solid fat.

I had a fortnight's holiday in February 1947 in the middle of my time at Dumfries and spent a week of it back in North Uist.

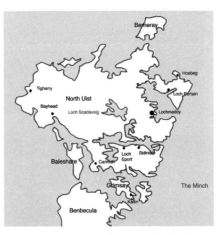

There, I did a few calls for Dr Macleod and escorted a patient with a miscarriage, in a motor boat across the Sound of Harris to Rodel, from where she went by ambulance to Stornoway.

It began to snow on the way back. It was the beginning of the 1947 snowstorms. I also went over to Lochportain in an open boat. The spray was freezing on us. It was cruel.

On my way back to Mallaig on the 'M.V. Lochmor', the cliffs on the island of Eigg had icicles several feet long, and from the West Highland Railway train I saw hundreds of deer driven off the mountains by the hard weather.

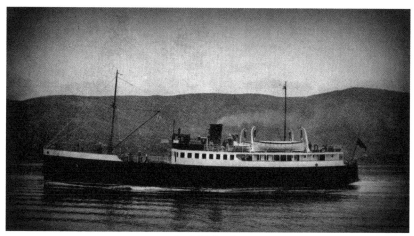
the MV Lochmor

All too soon, my eight day holiday in North Uist was over, and I was back to the routine of Dumfries Infirmary.

11. Not all work!

Mondays at Dumfries were 'tonsil days'. At that time, masses of children had their healthy tonsils removed, just because they were enlarged. So many children came in every week that they had to be put two in a bed – one at the top and one at the bottom.

On Tuesday afternoon there was a minor op. (operation) session. A lot of babies were brought in for circumcision. Of course, some were circumcised for religious reasons, but many parents just had their babies 'done', sometimes because it was a family tradition.

Some Wednesdays, Dr Fraser did eye operations. I was assisting one day when he asked me to raise the operating table with the foot pump. "That's not high enough!" he snapped. "Keep on until I tell you to stop!" Something distracted him and when he turned round the table was above eye level. I could be a bit of a mischief at times!

Mr Tom Millar came from Glasgow once a month to see outpatients and do some orthopaedic operations. He operated so fast it took two of us to give anaesthetics for him.

Sometimes, very ill patients had to be 'specialled' as they were recovering from an operation. This would be done in the recovery room of the theatre now. On one particular occasion, a boy was being watched by a nurse in a side ward. For some reason, I was there also and sat at the opposite side of the bed and fell for this nurse with her long dark eyelashes. (She lost these in later life when she developed Addison's disease.)

At Christmas, Mr Melrose, the elderly hospital chaplain, held a service in the ward at 10 am, when the doctors carved the turkey (a skill useful in later life!) There was carol singing round the wards in the evening. We had a party for Nurse Mills (who was leaving) in the duty room after the patients were settled. The food was all laid out when Matron arrived

25

unexpectedly but, thankfully, she did not go in. (Nurse Mills married a banker and died a few years ago at home in Denholm.) Later in the week, the ward maids had their party and the doctors did the serving.

Mention of Anne Mills reminds me of my second night at Dumfries. She was acting Sister in the operating theatre and a girl from Johnston Bridge was brought in having been run over by a tractor. She had serious abdominal injuries but survived. I wonder if she is still alive today. If so, she must be in her seventies.

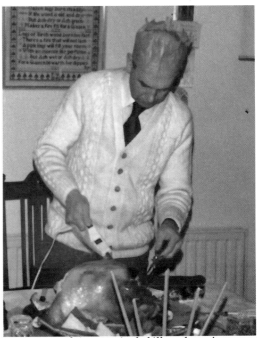

applying surgical skills at home!

12.   24th October 1946

Joyce (my future wife) described the events of 24th October, 1946:

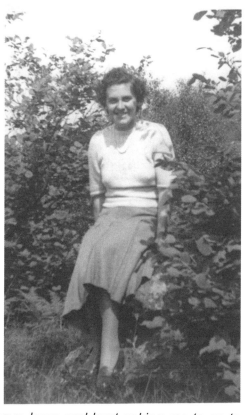

"As a baby, I was chosen by the White family of Papcastle, who already had four boys. I was brought up to go to Sunday School and church and to go the right way. I was christened in the Church of England and confirmed, though looking back I don't think I had any faith to confirm.

I always wanted to be a nurse, so at the age of 17½, I went to Dumfries Infirmary to train. In my year, there were four committed Christian nurses, who were keen and kept asking me to go to meetings. The evangelist Roy Hessian was holding a mission in Dumfries and these nurses wanted me to go to the afternoon ladies' meeting, but I had the perfect excuse – I was on night duty and would be in bed during the day.

That morning I went to bed but could not sleep. I got up and had a cup of tea, but still could not sleep, so I decided to get up and go for a walk. As I went out of the gate of Beechwood, the night nurses' home, who should be coming down the road but three of the nurses. "Oh, White, (that was my name) you're coming!"

I meekly followed!

At the end of the meeting, everyone left, but I was paralysed. I could not move, and Mrs. Hessian came and asked me if I wanted to trust Jesus as my Saviour. She prayed with me and I asked Jesus to come into my life and take control of it. It was wonderful: my sins were all forgiven. I was on my way to heaven.

Mrs. Hessian told me to tell others, so I told the other nurses who shared my room. I was due on duty at 9 pm, in charge of a 30-bedded male ward. I thought, "Who will I tell? I'll tell Dr. Bethune. He is a Christian. He'll be about the ward." I found, however, he was in a side room, ill!

After I had settled the other patients, I went into the side room. I told him, "Something wonderful happened to me today. I have trusted Jesus as my Saviour."

Mrs. Hessian had told me that other Christians would be glad when I told them, but he wept! He then explained that he had been in love with me for some time. He had made no advances, but had prayed for me."

This was the girl with the long dark eyelashes! (see p.25)

Two days later, she was moved from my ward to the medical ward. The timing was perfect. Soon we were going out. A year later we were engaged, and a wonderful 58 years marriage followed.

Of course, at that time, it was strictly forbidden for a nurse in training to have a relationship with any of the junior doctors. On the wards the nurses were called 'Nurse', the doctors 'Doctor' and the Sister 'Sister'. We knew many of the nurses by their Christian names but never in front of a patient. What a change today! One day when out together, we met the Matron, and Joyce was summoned to the office the next day, but somehow we managed to get away with it, perhaps because Joyce's training was nearly over.

Christmas Day was the only day when the rules were relaxed. You were in danger of being kissed by a nurse under the mistletoe! In fact, I trapped six nurses in the duty room and kissed each one under my piece of mistletoe as they came out. The last one was Joyce, with a face like a beetroot!

13. *Winter arrives*

On the first icy morning of the winter, there were seven elderly ladies outside the X-ray department. They *all* had fractured wrists, having walked out of their homes not realising how slippery the pavements were.

There was snow in February but the real winter snowstorm hit us on 12th March 1947. Dumfries was completely cut off until a train got through from Carlisle the next day. Dr Gordon Hunter got stuck in Kirkcudbright and had to walk to Crocketford, a distance of about 19 miles, to get back to Dumfries. One nurse who had been at home on her day off walked five miles to get back.

We suffered from bed-blocking. In an emergency, neighbours and roadmen made strenuous efforts to get the patient **to** hospital but there was no incentive to get recovered patients **back** to their snowbound homes. On one occasion, a patient developed chicken pox in the ward. It's so highly infectious we had to send him home. How?

We muffled him up and put him on the train!

Petrol was still rationed so we did not have the number of road accidents with which the modern hospitals have to deal.

We did have some, though. There were casualties from a bus accident in Maxwelltown. I remember specially a man with a fractured femur from a car crash at Johnstone Bridge on the A74. His fractured femur was fixed but the next day he complained of pains in his chest. X-ray revealed 12 broken ribs and I had given him an anaesthetic the day before.

Dumfries got all the casualties from the Ecclefechan train smash in July 1945. That strained the hospital's resources and I understand some mattresses were put on the floor for some casualties. Joyce was out with the ambulance that afternoon.

And here is a warning to anyone working on a saw bench. A man from Shawhead was cutting timber. A log jammed and he decided to kick it clear. The saw cut his leg off at mid-thigh. All we could do was to patch up the stump.

One night about midnight, a water-baillie was brought in, his clothes soaking. He had been struggling with a poacher who was using a salmon gaff. Both men had fallen into the River Cluden. Instead of a fish, the poacher gaffed the baillie. The thick gaff had passed through his arm above the wrist and miraculously under all the tendons without damaging them or any blood vessels. We wanted to keep the weapon, but the police took it away as evidence.

What other dramas did we have?

One nurse was being so harassed by the Ward Sister (not my ward) when she was cutting bread for the patients' suppers that she threatened the Sister with the bread knife. The Sister fled but the nurse was at the Matron's office next day.

Amputated limbs etc. were burned in the hospital furnace. One nurse was taking a leg over to be burned but had forgotten the key so went back for it. When she got back she was horrified to find that the leg she had left propped up beside the door was missing. By this time, an Alsatian dog was carrying it down St. Michael Street!

One lady arrived from horse jumping with a broken arm supported by an umbrella as a splint. We put a plaster on and sent her home, but during the night it became tight and two of us drove to the country beyond Lockerbie to take it off.

During the University vacation, we had students at the hospital. They stayed at the Grove convalescent home where Dr Gibson, the house physician, also lived. A hedgehog was found in the hospital grounds and as a prank they put it in Dr Gibson's bed, not realising it would make such a mess. He got his revenge by giving the Grove Staff Nurse (Joyce) some oil to put in the butter for the students' supper sandwiches. She did not realize that it was croton oil (a purgative for horses).

Needless to say, there was an outbreak of 'food poisoning' during the night.

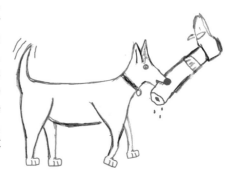

14. On to Cresswell Hospital

Nowadays, in the Cumberland Infirmary and the BGH, patients get a menu and select their meals for the next day, but in the old days the meals came up in bulk from the hospital kitchen and the ward sister or the staff nurse served it out onto individual plates. Often there was surplus and one evening a fellow house surgeon and I each ate three helpings of tripe left over in the female ward (and then went on to eat our own supper in the dining room).

Nellie, one of the older ward maids, fed her elderly friend Ned with left-overs. One evening, after a day off, Nellie told us she had been married that day as Ned was now 65 and had received his old age pension. Several years later, we saw them walking happily together beside the River Nith.

The summer of 1946 rolled on and my year at the Infirmary ended in early August. I had six weeks free until my next job at the Cresswell Counties Maternity Hospital in Dumfries – so called because it was funded mainly by the three Galloway County Councils, Dumfriesshire, the Stewartry and Wigtownshire.

Naturally I was off to North Uist again for a couple of weeks, doing some of Dr Macleod's visits on the island, but I managed an extended tour of the Outer Isles as well.

Meanwhile, Joyce had been accepted by the Baptist Missionary Society to go to China with me.

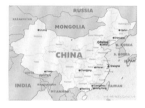

Her training as a nurse finished in October and, instead of going to Oswestry to train as an orthopaedic nurse as originally planned, went to the Elsie Inglis Hospital in Edinburgh to train as a midwife, as this would be more useful abroad. We got engaged two days before she left Dumfries. We didn't realise that it would be 3½ years before we got married.

Cresswell was a smaller hospital than the Infirmary, which had been purpose built as a hospital. Cresswell was an ex-poorhouse. There were two wards – an open Florence Nightingale type – and a private, paying ward with better facilities. The babies were kept in the nursery and brought along to their mothers only to be fed. At 6 am, a trolley full of crying babies rolled past the senior doctor's bedroom. An hour later the trolley rumbled back – not a sound – full of contented babies full of milk.

Dr Bruce Dewar was consultant in charge, with Dr Donald Beaton as his assistant. There were two house surgeons. The first three months I was junior house surgeon and for the next three months, senior house surgeon. The junior house surgeon had a cubicle in the nurses' corridor. That would have been unheard of in the Infirmary! The senior had a bed in our dining/sitting room. As the residency was mixed sex, we had our breakfasts in bed as the senior had to get up and dress in the common room.

For the first few weeks I was there, we had a water shortage. A new housing estate had been built after the war and we were at the end of the water main. The trouble was especially acute on Monday mornings – washing day. Often we had either hot or cold water, but not both. If you ran a hot bath you had to wait for it to cool down. One day we were so short of water that some nurses had to go and draw water from the wartime static water tank outside.

There was an open bar electric radiator in the operating theatre! The hospital lift was manually controlled. You got inside the lift alongside the trolley and pulled a heavy rope to move it up and down.

The standard of care, however, was very high and we had no problems with infections though, at that time, not being aware of the radiation dangers, every woman who came to the antenatal clinic for her first pregnancy had her pelvis X-rayed! Once a week, we had a conference with the Infirmary Radiologist, Dr McWhirter, to assess whether the shape of the pelvis might cause birth problems.

Dr Dewar came in to the hospital about 11 am each morning. If a patient was to be discharged that day, we had to have the case sheets completed and taken to the office before he came in. He went straight to the office and dictated a discharge letter. Before he left (about 1pm) he went back and signed the letters and they were in the hands of the GP the next morning.

15. More from Cresswell

On one of those beautiful sunny November mornings we sometimes get, Dr Beaton and I, with a bottle of blood, drove out to a farmhouse in the Glenkens area of Galloway in response to a call from Dr Carmichael of New Galloway. A patient of his had had a severe haemorrhage after childbirth. We gave her a blood transfusion, hanging the bottle of blood from the picture rail in the bedroom. Afterwards, Dr Carmichael took us for a meal at the Lochinvar Hotel in Dalry.

In February we had two hospital trips to Glasgow. Half of the staff went one week – Matron or assistant matron, sisters, nurses, ward maids and one house surgeon – and the other half the next week. We went to Glasgow on the morning train and returned by the 9.05 pm from St Enoch station (the night sleeper train to London).

We all met at the Alhambra Theatre for the pantomime in the afternoon, but otherwise we were free. In the evening, I went to the Western Infirmary to see my friend Tom Russell who had been a house surgeon at Dumfries after me.

Dumfries town had a small maternity unit called Charnwood. The patients from Dumfries town went there if their confinement was expected to be uncomplicated. They were normally looked after by their GPs, but we had to go there sometimes. It was a nice change, and the matron there made good coffee!

One morning Dr Dewar said, "Arthur, I have to go to Edinburgh for two days to examine candidates for the M.R.C.O.G. (the specialist degree in Obstetrics and Gynaecology). Dr Beaton is ill so I am leaving you in charge of the hospital."

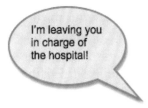

I'm leaving you in charge of the hospital!

"I will phone each evening to see if things are all right. If you are in real trouble, get Dr Milne from Carlisle!" He wasn't gone an hour when I had to deal with a complicated delivery, but I managed. No disasters!

At Cresswell, we did a trial of Pethidine as an analgesic

in labour. Dr Beaton wrote up the results and published them in a paper. It fell to me to do the statistics as he was no mathematician. Dr Beaton later became consultant at Dorchester. Cresswell was replaced a few years ago by a new unit beside the present infirmary. Sadly, I believe the old building has been demolished.

The junior doctor was up for every delivery. There was a ship's telegraph between his room and the labour ward. The senior doctor was not up so much, but was frequently called by phone during the night. This was much more trying, and by the end of March 1948 (when my six months was over), I was physically exhausted and had a serious worsening of my chronic genetic digestive problem. This was investigated by Dr J. D. S. Cameron (the best gastroenterologist in Edinburgh) and he gave me the news that going abroad was out of the question. The army did not want me either, so our lives (Joyce's and mine) were turned upside down.

So, what next?

Actually, about the same time, the BMS hospital in Taiyuanfu in North China to which I would have been appointed, was overrun by the advancing Communist army and the BMS staff had to be withdrawn.

During May, Mr Beveridge (my former boss at the Infirmary) asked me to go to Creetown for a few weeks as Dr George Hunter, the GP there, was going to hospital for investigation. Little did I know that this would extend to seven months. Dr Hunter was seriously ill and died in November aged only 35.

As I left home to catch the train, the postman handed me a letter. I opened it on the train to find it was from Dr Macleod asking me to return to Uist on a permanent basis. If I had received that letter a few days earlier my life might have been quite different, but God had a plan to lead both Joyce and myself to Newcastleton. North Uist was not in his plan. I never lost my love for North Uist, and Joyce and I often visited it on holiday.

During the seven months in Creetown, Joyce and I had only eight days together. She completed her midwifery training and stayed on at Elsie Inglis hospital as a Staff Midwife on the district attending many confinements in the poorer part of Edinburgh.

16. Creetown

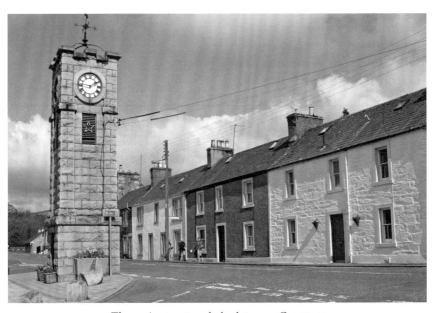

The main street and clock tower, Creetown

Creetown is a small town, 45 miles west of Dumfries on the Galloway coast and quite close to the sea. The practice, however, is not as extensive as the Newcastleton one, extending six miles west to the outskirts of Newton Stewart and eight miles east to Auchenlarie and Cardoness, both now well-known for their holiday caravan parks, with some farms up in the hills.

The doctor's house was unusual. A road ran steeply up past the side of the house, resulting in the first floor being on a level with the road. The bedrooms were upstairs, and at the far end of the corridor was the surgery with its own entrance onto the outside road. Some years later, when there were serious floods in Creetown, the flood water came in through the surgery door and poured through the house.

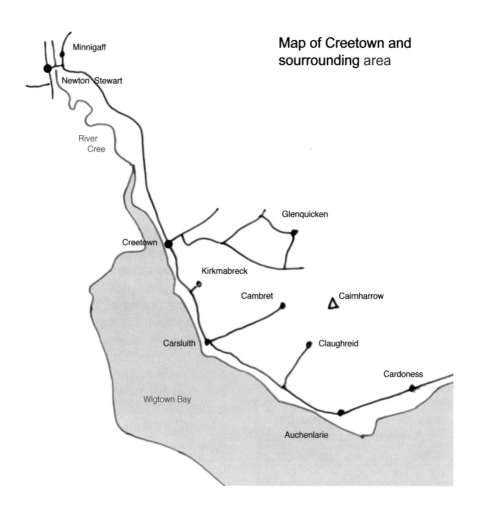

Map of Creetown and sourrounding area

The practice was non-dispensing. There was a chemist in the village and patients went to her for their repeat medicines. She kept a note of these and the doctor wrote up the prescriptions once a month so that, when the NHS started, she could submit them to the NHS for reimbursement.

On my way to Creetown, I visited my old ward at Dumfries Infirmary. The train connection was so bad I had four hours to wait at Dumfries. When I got to Creetown at 8 pm, I immediately sent a man with a perforated duodenal ulcer off to my old ward!

The granite quarry at Kirkmabreck was the main industry with a firm making concrete blocks etc, as a spin-off. I soon discovered that every wound contaminated with the granite became rapidly infected. Liverpool docks were constructed with Creetown granite.

One afternoon, a worker at the quarry sustained a fractured femur. The ambulance for the area was stationed at Kirkinner, eight miles south of Newton Stewart and 15 miles away. It had just left to take an emergency to Stranraer, where there was a hospital with a GP surgeon which dealt with minor surgery. We took the patient home on the back of a lorry and he was collected by the ambulance over two hours later.

There are two farms, Cambret and Claughreid, each over two miles into the hills with numerous gates. Claughreid had six. The farms were seven miles apart by road, but less than a mile apart directly. If I had to visit both, I usually walked from one to the other, once climbing a hill, Cairnharrow, on the way.

One afternoon at 2 pm, I was doing rounds when I remembered I had put a thermometer under a patient's arm in the forenoon but forgot to take it out. I hurried back to the farm cottage. The thermometer was still under his arm where I had left it three hours before and, amazingly, intact.

Actually, I rarely used a thermometer during my career as a doctor.

The doctor's maid / receptionist left to marry the local butcher, so they employed another young lady who was not local. One night, she answered the phone and told me there was a call for Weir Cottage, Carsluith, where a boy was bleeding after coming home from hospital where he had had his tonsils removed. It was the middle of the night. She didn't know where the cottage was. Neither did I – so I set off for Carsluith looking for a house with a light on. No luck! I contacted the local Post Office by phone and was told that the cottage was down a long footpath beside the sea. No wonder I could not see a light.

Fortunately the bleeding had stopped by the time I eventually got there. Later, I found it was easier to walk along the seashore from another road to reach the cottage.

In a holiday cottage nearby, I encountered the boy whose appendix had been removed when his hernia was repaired (mentioned in chapter 10). It reminded me that Mr Beveridge (Dumfries surgeon), when on holiday at Arisaig, saw a boy with a surgery scar on his abdomen and discovered he had operated on the boy as a baby, for pyloric stenosis.

The NHS started on 5th July 1948. My last private visit was to a lady who sent for me at 11pm the night before. She had to pay for her visit, but I gave her an NHS prescription form so she got the medicine the next morning. I expect it was technically illegal to give an NHS form to a private patient.

We sent out the outstanding bills, but less than a third paid. After Dr Hunter died in November, the accounts were sent out again, only this time they were payable to the lawyer who was winding up Dr Hunter's affairs. The money came flooding in. I think patients thought they were going to be sued for payment!

17. From Creetown back to Edinburgh

While I was at Creetown, there was a violent thunderstorm. At Glenquicken farm, the farmer's mother-in-law was baking. The lightning struck the chimney and blew a chip out of the wooden baking board. She was unhurt but, understandably, a bit shaken.

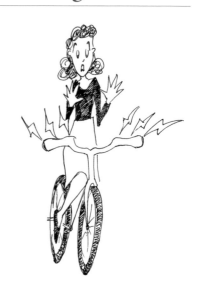

The daughter of the farmer at Claughreid was cycling home. On the way, there was lightning and she got a slight electric shock from the handlebars.

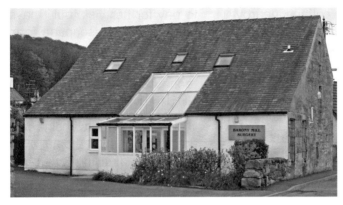

The Creetown Health Centre, in 2012 - no longer in the doctor's house!

During my time there, two sets of twins and one set of triplets were born. Sadly, a 40-year mother lost her first baby. I was called too late. The baby had already died.

I came across a disease new to me – Bornholm's Disease – so called because it was first described on the island of Bornholm in the Baltic. It is caused by the Coxsackie virus. The patient is feverish and gets severe localised pain in the abdominal and chest muscles. It can mimic many serious illnesses – appendicitis, gall bladder inflammation and pleurisy. In the chest, it is known as 'The Devil's grip'.

The practice was single-handed, so you were on call all the time, but there was an arrangement with Dr Kellie Brooke of Minigaff to cover emergencies on Wednesday afternoon and evening each week – the practice half day. On one of these, I went to hear Prof. Derrick Dunlop lecture on a new family of drugs: the anti-histamines. These are the drugs used for allergic conditions like hay fever and urticaria (hives).

Going to Kirkmabreck Parish Church one morning I got a big surprise. The young preacher was Robin Wallace who had been in my class at school. I had never seen or heard of him since leaving school. He was a native of Creetown. Later, he became Church of Scotland minister in Carlisle and then in Brydekirk, near Annan.

It was at Creetown that I made my first contact with the Christian Brethren. I had thought them to be dull, spoil-sport people, but found them bright, friendly and happy.

At Creetown, I attended a young woman in a real gipsy caravan. Crossways, in the back of the van, there was a normal bed in which the patient was lying. Her mother, Gipsy Lee, told me my fortune (not very exciting). That was the only payment I got as they did a midnight flit and were gone when I went back the next day.

Dr Hunter died in November and his widow kept the practice going to the end of the year. I decided to go back to hospital work and had an interview for a job at Alder Hey Hospital in Liverpool but did not get it, so on January 3rd 1949, I left Creetown with no job in prospect.

However, a senior house officer's job turned up at the Astley Ainslie Hospital in Edinburgh, so I started there on 1st February. It was a fairly easy job with time to study for a further degree. That was the plan!

The Astley Ainslie was a convalescent hospital for the Edinburgh Royal Infirmary. I was in charge of two medical wards (one male, one female). The patients were mostly recovering from rheumatic fever, common in those days, and with the potential to develop rheumatic heart disease, or were recovering from pleurisy with effusion, suspected, but not proven, tuberculosis. They had sanatorium treatment and the beds were often out on the verandas if the weather allowed. The doctors found it cold. Try taking off blood with white fingers!

It was at the Astley Ainslie that I saw the only case of diphtheria I have ever seen. It was in a child who had been in hospital for some time. A visitor must have carried the infection in. Actually, by that time, diphtheria had been almost eradicated by immunisation. The child made a good recovery.

It was here I came across bureaucracy in the NHS for the first time. We had a rota listing the doctors on duty in the hospital. To swap duties, we had to apply in triplicate to the Superintendent. He was an ex-army colonel!

The assistant superintendent was Jimmy Sommerville. I knew him well as he had been two years ahead of me at school and we had both belonged to the Field Club, a natural history society.

He told me how he had worked for Prof. Learmouth, professor of surgery, who had operated on King George VI.

One day, the Professor was operating at Gogarburn Hospital a few miles out of Edinburgh. He amputated a leg and told Jimmy to take it to the Dept. of Surgery laboratory at the University. Jimmy had no car, but you didn't argue with "the Prof".

He wrapped the leg up, then thumbed a lift on the A8. The driver kept looking at the parcel.

"That's a strange parcel!"

"Yes".

"It looks awfully like a leg!"

"It is a leg", said Jimmy.

With that, the driver said: "We're at the Corstorphine tram terminus, so I'll let you off."

18. First contact with Newcastleton

At the Astley Ainslie Hospital, the doctors' residence was about a quarter of a mile from my wards, so I used my bicycle to and fro. There were two other residents – Ruth Armitage and Alastair Kingsley Brown. The latter became a Harley Street consultant. Ruth was not allowed to sleep in the residency. She had a bedroom in the office block. It would not have been 'proper' for her to sleep in the residency, although we were all senior doctors by then.

One day, I was with the radiologist who was doing a barium swallow X-ray. The patient drank mouthfuls of the barium mixture and we watched on the X-ray screen as it went down the oesophagus and into his stomach. It was dark in the room. Suddenly, the live X-ray picture vanished. A power cut? No! After about two seconds there was a thud. The patient had fainted and collapsed on the floor. Miraculously he was unharmed.

The lab technician at the hospital had a narrow escape. He had bad indigestion and kept a jar of magnesium trisilicate on his work bench. One day, he took a spoonful and realised to his horror he had taken sodium fluoride by mistake. Fluorides are used to etch glass. If he hadn't been in hospital he would not have survived, but he was left with a very distorted oesophagus and stomach.

The Astley Ainslie housed the Occupational Therapy training school. One of my patients was a scientist who was studying 'Neurosis in ants' (*ants* not *aunts!*) I cannot imagine the use of such a study.

1949 was a glorious summer and my fiancée was working in Edinburgh so the intended study for another degree got sidetracked. On 20th May, we walked over Blackford Hill and made the momentous decision that my future lay in general practice.

So, I started looking for a permanent job and found one at Ibstock in Leicestershire.

Joyce continued as a district midwife in Edinburgh, but a few months later her mother took seriously ill, and she went home to Papcastle and never returned to Edinburgh. She attended many confinements in the poorer and rougher areas in central Edinburgh and could go, alone, anywhere in safety. At that time, nurses, midwives and Salvation Army lassies could go on their own and in safety, on streets in which policemen ventured only in pairs.

Many of the stairways were dark, having no lighting. One night she had to send for the doctor and, on answering the door, all she could see were his two eyes.

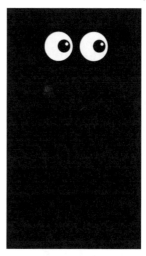

The doctor was black and his suit dark coloured!

Some houses had beds in the kitchen and the coal cellar was also there. (In fact, when I was small we had a bed and the coal cellar in the kitchen). At one confinement, the husband did not want to see what was happening, so he spent the time with his head in the coal cellar doorway!

For some time, Joyce had to live at the District Nurses' Training school. The lights were put out at 10 pm so, if she was late in from a case, it was dark and there was no food. The taxi drivers at Croall's garage across the road used to share their sandwiches with her.

I had six weeks to go before the Ibstock job started and I went one day to the British Medical Association office about insurance.

The secretary said:

Dr Murdoch of Newcastleton has just phoned in for a locum for 4 weeks. You are free. Will you go?

I was in Newcastleton by 2 pm the next afternoon!

That is how I made my first contact with the village.

A year before I had passed through on the evening train from Carlisle and, as the train passed the Muckle Knowe, had looked up the long wide street with the Congregational Church spire, not dreaming I would spend my life there.

I had also been through the village in the train twice on my way to interviews for jobs in Leicestershire.

Chance? Luck?   No!

It was all God's plan and perfect timing to bring Joyce to Newcastleton to do such wonderful work among the Guides and the Old Age Pensioners and the local church.

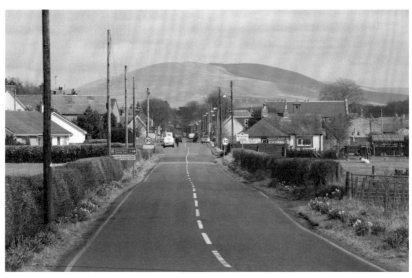

"Looking up the long wide street" in 2013, the Congregational Church spire now replaced by a bell tower, but with Arnton Fell still dominating the view

19.   A place called Newcastleton

In the last quarter of the 19th century there were two doctors in Newcastleton – Dr T. C. Taylor and his son James. They lived and practised from 5 Douglas Square. About 1894, a new doctor arrived, Dr Rufus Evans. I suspect Dr Taylor Snr. was failing in health then, as he died in 1903 aged 74. Dr James Taylor died in 1921, and must have practised to the end as there were 1921 clinical records with his name when I came here. He is reported to have had a steam car. It took three hours to raise steam – not very useful in an emergency – and required a mechanic from Manchester for repairs!

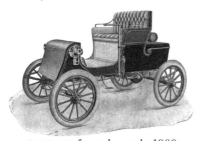

a steam car from the early 1900s

Dr Evans lived at Park Villa (now Castleton Manse, but then a Temperance Hotel) and had a surgery at Scott's the bakers. Later, he married Rose Vassie, the sister of the minister of Castleton Church, and he built Northfield, where he practised until his retirement in 1942. His retirement presentation was held in the Mechanics Hall (now the British Legion) and it was chaired by Simon Bell, the stationmaster, grandfather of the well-known broadcaster, Eric Robson.

Dr J.M. Stewart took over from Dr Evans in 1942 and practised from Dr Taylor's old house, but he moved to Largo in Fife in 1945. Dr James Murdoch, who married Dr Evans' daughter Mary, took over and the surgery returned to Northfield.

So, when I arrived in Newcastleton on 25th August 1949 as a locum, it was Jimmy Murdoch who met me at the station. After dumping my belongings at Northfield, we did a round of visits up Liddel Water and down Hermitage. My first patients were Bet Semple's mother, and daughter Lily, at Byreholm. I also visited the Aitchisons in Hermitage Cottage.

Next day, Mrs Murdoch took me round Penton and Bewcastle, and introduced me to Mrs Emily

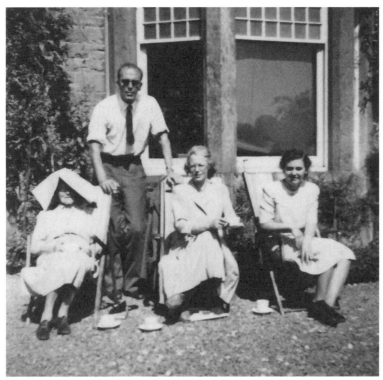

Mrs Evans, Dr and Mrs Murdoch and Joyce
in the front garden of Northfield, 1950

Lauder at Roughsyke, where we had a 'house of call'. Patients could come there at 2 pm on Tuesdays and Fridays. My first patient in Bewcastle was the late Sadie Graham of Kershopefoot. She was at her mother's house at Craigyford before she and her husband settled in Carlisle.

Then the Murdochs went off on their holiday and left Mary Murdoch's sister, Helen Rhys, in charge. Helen is better known as the historical novelist Jane

Oliver. Her husband had been a pilot and was killed in the Battle of Britain. Helen drove ambulances in the London Blitz. For staff, there was Peggy Hyslop, the cook, and 'Chip' Little, who did the cleaning. Eva Cowan came every Monday to do the week's washing.

Only those over 60 will remember the surgery at the back of the house. At surgery times, patients came in by the front door and waited in the dining room. Sometimes we were disturbed at breakfast by early arrivals. If you came at any other time, you would be entertained by Peggy in the kitchen until the doctor was available.

After your consultation, you left the surgery by a direct door out to the back. The dispensary for drugs was half of the adjacent domestic pantry. The drugs came from T&H Smith of Edinburgh by goods train and were delivered from the station by horse and cart. They were packed in straw in tea-boxes and we emptied them in the garage to avoid a mess in the house. There was a 5/- (25p) deposit on each box, and it was worthwhile to send the boxes back to Edinburgh at the 'Returned Empties' charge to

get the deposit back!

Soon, I had my first visit to Riccarton Junction, the railway village with no road. Coming back, Mr Gillies the station master took the engine (a Shire class) off the Newcastle train standing there and sent me down on the footplate.

It was 10 days before I went to Kielder. We had very few patients there then, as most of Castle Drive and all of Buttery Haugh was yet to be built.

My first contact there was Jock Scott, the postman, brother of Julie Cuthbert's granny, and my first visit was to The Forks, a mile up the Lewis Burn. By a strange coincidence my last visit to Kielder at my retirement 36 years later, was also to The Forks.

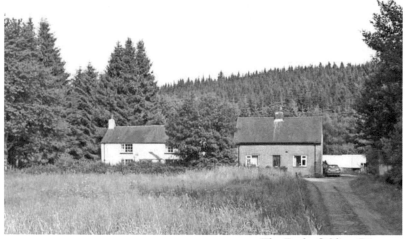

The Forks ©OliverDixon

I also experienced the only time I got lost in Bewcastle. Going up to visit the Carruthers family at Oakstocks, I was sent up the road just past Bewcastle church. "It's the first house you come to."

After two miles of rough road and three fords I arrived at High Grains. Oakstocks was 1¾ miles back!

How did I miss it?

Well, my informant failed to tell me the house was down a bank off the road and all you could see from the road was one chimney pot!

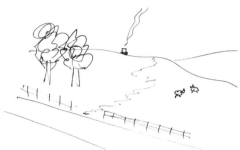

20. Off to Leicestershire

With a wave from Mr Gillies on the platform at Riccarton Junction and a brief view of Newcastleton, on the first day of October 1949, I passed through Liddesdale on the Waverley express on my way to Ibstock in Leicestershire, where I anticipated spending the rest of my working life.

The medical practice which I was joining was based in the large village of Ibstock (we would consider it a small town in Scotland) on the edge of the North West Leicestershire coalfield.

Despite there being four active collieries in the practice area, it was quite a rural setting.

There were a dozen villages scattered around, none more than five miles away. Three had obviously developed with the coal industry, but the others were typical old English villages, developing round the Parish Church.

All the houses were accessible by road – quite a change for me!

Six miles away was the old unspoiled town of Market Bosworth, where there was a small hospital – Market Bosworh Park Infirmary, formerly the Manor house. Here, Joyce got an appointment as a Sister.

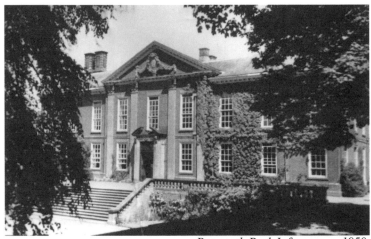

Bosworth Park Infirmary, c. 1950

The hospital catered for quite a mix of patients – maternity, tonsillectomies and a ward for disabled children. One day, Joyce had to deliver a baby in a taxi in the hospital car park. The taxi driver was not amused! The hospital is now a hotel and Joyce and I spent a weekend there eleven years ago.

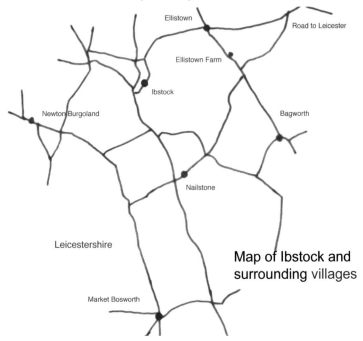

Map of Ibstock and surrounding villages

There were two doctors. Walter Meldrum, an Orcadian, had been there a long time. His son, Keith, became Chief Veterinary Officer at the time of the BSE crisis.

The other was Arthur Watts, who had spent some time in South Africa and whose father had been rector of Nailstone Church nearby.

Morning surgery started at 8.30 am, but Dr Watts had a special interest in psychiatry and he saw a psychiatric case by appointment at 8am each morning. At first, patients were slow to come to the new young doctor and I whiled away some of the time reading A J Cronin's novels, but soon people realised it was safe to come to me!

Dr Watts had a peripheral surgery and visits at Bagworth village (three miles away). He retained the prescription forms as he went round and in the early afternoon, Mr Restall, the chemist, tracked him down and had the medicines made by early evening, when a man came from Bagworth, collected the medicines and delivered them to patients for a fee of 1/- (5p) each.

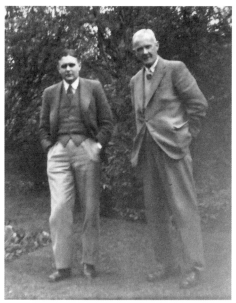

Dr Watts and Dr Meldrum, Ibstock, 1950

Medically, we had all the normal illnesses but, being a mining area, a high incidence of chronic chest diseases and bad backs, also 'beat knees' bursitis from kneeling at the coalface, and miners' nystagmus, an eye problem caused by long periods in poor lighting.

A man with heart trouble was in a bus which had to make an emergency stop. He was thrown forward and the diseased aortic valve of his heart was completely ruptured. He died in 36 hours. Only cardiac surgery could have saved him, but of course it was not available then.

I was horrified one day to see a man with gangrene of both hands, brought on by the vibrations of a pneumatic road drill.

Another day, in an isolated country cottage, a patient, whom I attended quite often, threatened me with a bread knife. I kept the kitchen table between us and talked her out of the problem.

I had 'digs' at Ellistown farm, two miles away. Mrs Grainger, the farmer's wife, went to all the local pig killings and made Melton Mowbray pork pies, for which Leicestershire is famous. I ate masses of those pies while I was there. They were good – better than Walker's famous pies.

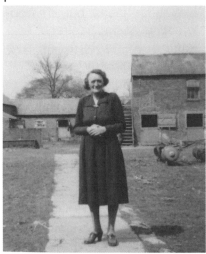

Mrs Grainger, my landlady at Ellistown Farm

There are two other Newcstleton connections with Ibstock. Alec Nichol has planted trees there and Rev. Idris Vaughan (former Minister of the Congregational Church) had been Congregational Minister at one of the villages – Newton Burgoland.

One of the attractions to me was the local Baptist church, of which I became a member. The church secretary and his wife became lifelong friends.

I was offered a partnership in the practice but there was no house available. The only answer was to buy land and build a house, but this was financially impossible for me. Also, there were too many patients on the practice list and I found my standard of work was dropping – 'shoddy' I described it in my diary.

Dr James Murdoch offered me a permanent job here at Newcastleton, so on 30th April 1950, my 27th birthday, Joyce and I packed all our worldly possessions into my car and we left Leicestershire. I dropped Joyce at her home at Papcastle next day, and came on to Copshawholm, where I have lived ever since.

Disappointing that the job at Ibstock did not turn out as we had hoped? Yes! I am sure it must have been much worse for Joyce. Marriage seemed further away than ever. But it was all part of God's plan to lead me here just in time for the unexpected crisis in the practice four months later.

21. 1950, a year of change

Summer 1950 was a happy one. Jimmy Murdoch and I got on well. Most evenings after surgery, we walked to Whithaugh Pool and along the river to Pathhead.

The Murdochs, after five years of marriage, were expecting their first baby in November. Petrol rationing had ended and Joyce had obtained employment as a midwife at the Haig Maternity Hospital in Hawick. All we had to wait for now was a house to live in to turn up.

Jimmy told me some of his amusing experiences – how a patient had swallowed powders meant for his greyhounds (to no ill-effect!) and how he had been called to a motorbike accident as the driver had broken his leg. It turned out to be his wooden leg that was broken! Just as the severe 1947 snowstorm started, he told a patient in an isolated cottage to stay in bed till he came back. They were snowed up for some time so he thought the relatives would get the man up. Six weeks later he received an SOS. "When are you coming back? We are having a job keeping him in bed."

But in August, Jimmy did not seem to be well and, as he was getting worse, I took him to Carlisle on 9th September for an X-ray. The seriousness of his condition was confirmed, and two days later he was admitted to Shotley Bridge Hospital. After his discharge from hospital, he and Mary went to stay with his sister, Mrs Torrance, at Shotts.

The result was I was left to run the practice alone, which I was to do for the next 13 months with some intermittent assistance. First, for six weeks in Jan / Feb, by Dr Andrew Douglas, who later became a chest consultant in Edinburgh, then for four weeks in June and two weeks in the autumn by Dr Grant McIntosh. Otherwise I did every surgery, every night and weekend on call, all the dispensing (including the ordering of drugs) and dealing with all the paper work. Thankfully, it was only a fraction of what it is today. Indicative of the pressure I was under was that the almost daily diary I had kept since I was 11, ceased on 19th September.

Often, I was making up medicines at 9pm, ready to go out to the country next morning. Jim Cuthbert came up before school and distributed the various medicines to the Post Office and the shops. The post was sorted at the local post office and, for a fee of two pence (1p) the medicines were delivered by the mail. Beyond the local postal zone, medicines were carried by the grocer's and the butcher vans – R Oliver & sons, T&A Oliver, Carruthers & Scott, T Elliot & Son and the Co-op. There were vans going most places each day.

Medicines for Riccarton Junction went up free on the train, labelled 'On Company Service'!

In January 1951 I purchased 34, North Hermitage Street, which Sandy Scott the plumber had renovated before he decided to emigrate to Canada. Joyce handed in her notice, and seven weeks later (17th March), I managed a weekend off (Fri – Sun evening) to get married at Horwich in Lancashire.

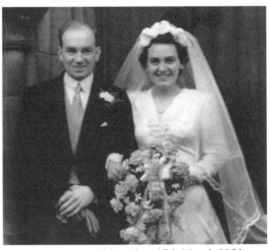

wedding day, 17th March 1951

We spent our first night at the Langdale Chase. As we walked into Northfield the next evening, to report to Peggy that we were back, the telephone rang to say that Dr Murdoch had died.

Next morning, my first visit was to Riccarton Junction where Mrs Gascoigne had died.

Some start to married life!

I had been promised a partnership but, on account of Jimmy's illness, nothing had been signed up. I expected the NHS would honour this but 'No', I had to apply for the practice and was interviewed along with two other candidates. The stress was not eased by the fact that a young doctor in a similar situation in Dundee had been passed over and the practice awarded to someone else. Anyway, I was appointed and took over the practice on 1st June,1951.

But where to have a surgery? No. 34 had only two bedrooms.

Zena Weir, Nicol Elliot's mother, came to the rescue. She let me have a front room at Fairview as the consulting room. She was a widow, struggling to bring up three children and badly needed the income.

The McIntoshes came for a month, helped with the transfer of everything from Northfield to Fairview, and then let Joyce and me off for our delayed honeymoon.

We had a wonderful two weeks based in Fort William.

We climbed Ben Nevis.

We sailed round Mull and landed at Iona and Fingal's Cave on Staffa.

We motored down the Ardnamurchan peninsula.

We sailed on the steamer from Mallaig round the Small Isles (Eigg, Rhum and Canna) and we caught up with old friends in Dalwhinnie and Inverness.

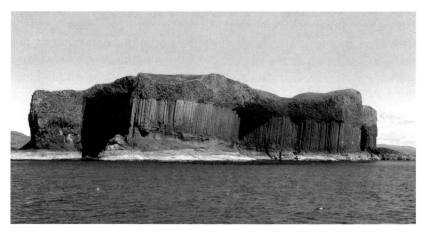

Staffa and Fingal's Cave

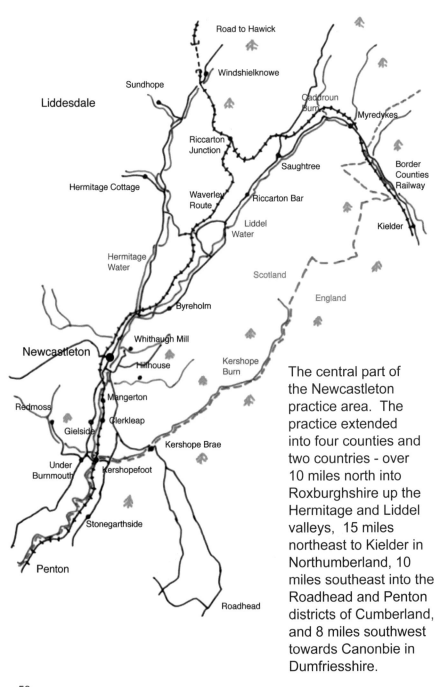

The central part of the Newcastleton practice area. The practice extended into four counties and two countries - over 10 miles north into Roxburghshire up the Hermitage and Liddel valleys, 15 miles northeast to Kielder in Northumberland, 10 miles southeast into the Roadhead and Penton districts of Cumberland, and 8 miles southwest towards Canonbie in Dumfriesshire.

22. *Getting the practice going*

I had been appointed to the practice and found surgery premises, but I needed money to buy the stock of drugs and the other medical equipment required. The NHS would pay me only every 3 months in arrears and there was no help with the surgery rent or ancillary help. Joyce and I had only £5 left in the bank after we set up house. Mr Learmouth, manager of the British Linen Bank (as it was then), stepped in and arranged a temporary overdraft facility.

The next item on the programme was to find an assistant to help me, and I found one in a pleasant, young, good Irish doctor – Wilfred Sinclair – who came in October 1951. He had 'digs' with Zena Elliot. He might well have stayed permanently but, though there was no National Service in Northern Ireland, after two years residence in Scotland, he was liable for National Service here. He chose to do this as a doctor in the Colonial Medical Service in Nyasaland (now Malawi) and subsequently settled in British Columbia. He settled well into village life, playing bowls and teaching in the Congregational Church Sunday School.

There were two major incidents during his time here. Every fourth weekend, he went home to Stewartstown in Ireland. On only one occasion did he change the weekend. Otherwise, he would have been on the Stranraer-Larne steamer, the Princess Victoria, when it sank with much loss of life in the severe gale of 1953.

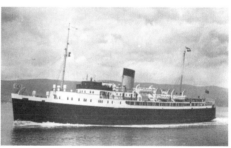

Princess Victoria

Wilfred Sinclair was engaged to a lady doctor – Olive Russell. Her parents had a pig farm in Co. Tyrone. Olive and Wilfred were getting married after Wilfred left here and she came to stay for a few days on her way home from Bacup, Lancashire, where she had been working as a GP. They went to Edinburgh to do some shopping and, after Olive went off home, we had word that a patient with whom she had been in contact in Bacup had developed smallpox. All her contacts here, and in the shops which they had visited in Edinburgh, had to be vaccinated. Olive was quarantined at home a week before her marriage. I am glad to say that the wedding took place as planned.

Wilfred was followed by a 6'4" Scotsman, Alex Watt. He worked here for three years, then went off to work in Lagos, Nigeria. He had two small children, and Mr David Oliver, County Councillor, was instrumental in getting him a 'keyworker's house' in the newly completed Oliver Place. There was an accident during the construction of those houses - a workman was trapped in a fall of earth in a trench. Fortunately, he was not seriously injured.

It was during Alex Watt's time that an RAF plane crashed into the hillside near Ettleton Cemetery. The pilot was killed instantly.

The pilot was only 19 and the only son of a widow. The plane passed over me near The Ash, Roadhead. The engines had cut out by then. Archie McKay came as part of the army guard, married local girl Jenny Maxwell and settled here on de-mob.

The Roxburgh Executive Council, the committee running the GP service, was administered part-time from Mr James Scott's accountant's office in Hawick. The district nurse was responsible directly to the Chief Nursing Officer. There was no Borders General Hospital then. All cases went to the Cumberland Infirmary in Carlisle. Peel Hospital, near Galashiels, was a small hospital which opened in 1939 as an Emergency Hospital for wartime.

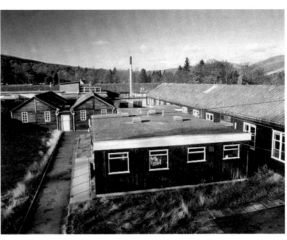

Peel Hospital

Though we did not send patients there, Peel played a significant part in my early life. My sister, Marion, was the first house physician there. I went several times and spent holidays at The Nest, the angling club B&B nearby, and often wandered about the hospital and the wards! I was still a schoolboy!

It could not happen today! It was there I got my desire to do medicine. Before that I was dead set on a career in mathematics. However, maths was my main subject in the Edinburgh University Bursary Competition and enabled me to gain a bursary to go to university and become a doctor.

23. *Riccarton Junction*

Locals who are over 40 will remember Riccarton Junction being occupied. It was the junction where the railway line from Hexham joined the Waverley route. There were about 30 houses for railway workers, the school and

schoolhouse, and two nearby properties – The Glen, down the hill below the station, and Phaupknowe, a shepherd's cottage ¼ mile away. We had 77 patients there and the Hawick doctors also had some.

Riccarton Junction c.1910
(from Bill Lynn collection)

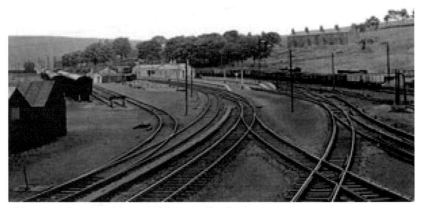

Riccarton Junction (from Bill Lynn collection)

There was no road access, the nearest road being two miles away, so we travelled there by train. Normally, we travelled up on the 8 am school train, which gave us an hour before catching the 9.25 train back to "The Holm". Many a time I have run down the hill and over the footbridge with the train standing in the station being held back for me by the Stationmaster.

In an emergency, we travelled by anything that was going - passenger train, goods train, or light engine sent specially down for us. We had 1st class passes for the passenger trains and special permits to travel in the brake van or on the footplate with the engine crew (see next page). We preferred travelling on the engine.

At first, I found it a strange feeling to be heading into the dark with no headlights, just trusting that the rails were there – rather like the Christian faith. If there was a late visit, I went up on the 8 pm train. Afterwards I would wait in the South Signal Box for transport home, usually on the St Boswell's goods.

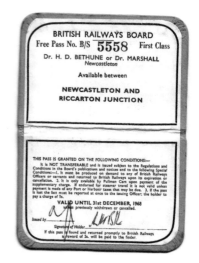

BRITISH RAILWAYS

THE RAILWAY EXECUTIVE
SCOTTISH REGION

T. F. CAMERON
CHIEF REGIONAL OFFICER
T. H. MOFFAT
DEPUTY CHIEF REGIONAL OFFICER
TELEPHONE:
DOUGLAS 2800. EXT.

302, BUCHANAN STREET,
GLASGOW, C.2.

E.R.O. 30951

The Bearer. Dr. Arthur D. Bethune of Northfield, Newcastleton,

is authorised to travel free in the Brake Vans of Goods and

Mineral Trains between Newcastleton and Riccarton Junction

subject to the terms of the Indemnity given by him in

respect of this permission.

Issued ....

Chief Regional Office,
302 Buchanan Street,
Glasgow, C.2.

27th March, 1951.

This Permit must be produced and given up when required.

33545 BRITISH TRANSPORT COMMISSION   B.R. 87103

British Railways....Scottish Region.5th. Feb.19.63.

Footplate and Driving Compartment Pass

The Bearer ..... DOCTOR BETHUNE

is authorised to ride

Upon		in the driving compartment of	
Steam		Diesel	
Diesel Main Line	Locomotives		Trains
Diesel Shunting		Electric	
Electric Main Line	(Rear cab only)		

.... train from ....

Between ..... Newcastleton

and ..... Hawick and return.

Until/~~by~~ ..... 31st December, 1963.
(Delete as necessary)

Issued for the B.T.C. by ....

This pass must be exhibited when required and is issued subject to
the conditions printed on the other side.

(FOR B.T.C. PERSONNEL)

58

One night the Edinburgh-London night express was stopped for me.

Engine driver Albert Snowdon, 'the mad man from the Tyne' they called him, was notorious for his fast driving.

He tried to frighten me one day, going backwards in under 10 minutes with a stop at Steele Road. The coal was tumbling out of the tender, the fire shovels were everywhere but I did not bat an eye and he never tried it again.

Going up with Albert another day (the driver of the Newcastle train had collapsed), he was going so fast that the locomotive actually rocked at the bend south of Steele Road.

On Sundays, there were no trains, so we walked in from Whitrope along the track. One day when there was a northerly gale, Joyce dropped me at Whitrope and I walked through to Saughtree Church, where she picked me up nearly two hours later.

On another occasion, during a railway strike, only one train ran. I went up with it and then walked out to Shaws Farm.

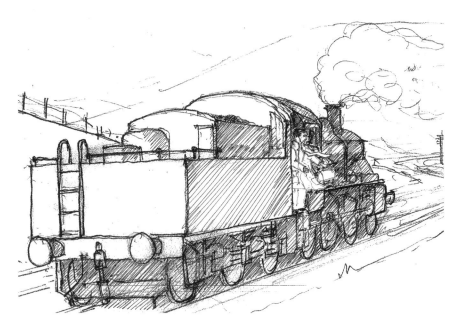

Albert Snowdon attempts to scare the doctor!

Clerkleap was another place which you reached by walking along the railway track. One night, we had to take a patient from Clerkleap to hospital, and Rob Wilson's father drove the platelayer's trolley down the line to Kershopefoot and picked us up on the way back. That was done quite illegally without control in Edinburgh knowing anything about it and not being recorded in the signal box log books.

On another occasion, as I walked back to Mangerton from Clerkleap, the local goods train pulled up. Driver Jim Wood looked out. "Do you want a lift to the Holm?" At a later date, Jim would allow me to drive the pilot engine from Riccarton to Newcastleton.

Emergencies from Riccarton had to be evacuated by passenger train. During the severe winter of 1963 when the line was blocked by snow north of Riccarton, we had to take a seriously ill patient to Newcastleton in the goods brake van, where she was transferred to an ambulance. She must have been very cold. There were no helicopters available then.

One foggy night I was going across the complicated junction pointwork to board the St Boswells goods when it went off into the fog without me. About 10 minutes later, the fireman appeared. The guard had put on the brakes, fearful I had fallen under the train, and stopped the train.

On another day with Albert, the pressure gauge on my side broke. Albert quickly smothered it with a cloth and switched it off.

This brings me to some of the hazards of general practice. One was sitting on a 'jammy piece' in a house in Riccarton.

Another was getting my car out to find a cat had used the driving seat as a toilet.

Only twice have I been attacked by dogs - small ones. Twice Alsatians have run away from me!

Tosh Mullans had a nasty bubbly jock (turkey) at the Nook, but Mrs Mullans kept a broom at the door for me to fight it off.

More seriously, twice angry patients have tried (unsuccessfully) to run me over!

24. More major changes

Dr Watt's departure to Nigeria coincided with Dr Grant McIntosh's return from Belgian Congo where he had been a medical missionary since his short time at Newcastleton. His return to Congo was delayed because of the political unrest following independence, and he came here until he could see the way ahead. That turned out to be three years.

The practice was now facing more problems. 34 North Hermitage Street was becoming too small for my expanding family. Zena Weir had re-married and naturally wanted the surgery away from her house. The problem was finding suitable property in the village.

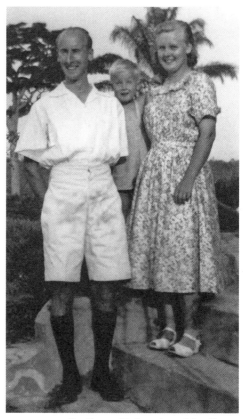

Dr Grant McIntosh and family while in Belgian Congo.

We made negotiations for both Whisgills and Woodside, but they were withdrawn from the market after we had them surveyed. We made an offer for Park Villa (now Castleton Manse). The church offered exactly the same amount but they increased their offer to well above the market value.

So, we made the decision to build a home, and made an offer for the field beside Holmhead and had plans drawn for a house with attached surgery premises.

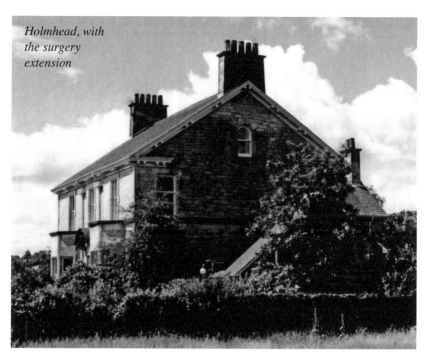

Holmhead, with the surgery extension

Meanwhile, Holmhead came on the market. We made an offer and it was accepted. Soon after that, our offer for the field was also accepted, but we were not bound by it as the closing date had been five months earlier. We built the side entrance and consulting room onto the house. The surgery premises were quite advanced for the time.

It was in that surgery some years later, that I would kneel and ask Jesus into my life. Since a Scripture Union meeting when I was 13, I had been convinced of the truth of the Christian faith – our need for salvation – forgiveness of sins by trusting in the sacrifice of Jesus Christ on Calvary - but it was all head knowledge. Now, my life was committed and I entered a totally new life.

And that's where the surgery remained until my retiral in 1985, when the new Dr Blair moved into Holmhead and the surgery moved to 4 South Liddel Street.

Dr McIntosh returned temporarily to Congo in 1960 where he was captured and almost shot, only to be saved by the intervention of an officer who recognised him.

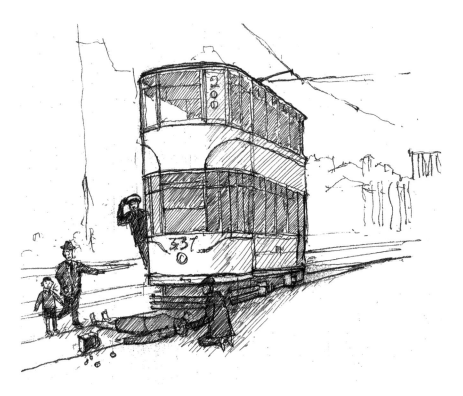

Mention of Dr McIntosh reminds me that, on the evening before my graduation, we were walking up Lothian Road in Edinburgh when there was a loud clatter. A drunk man had been bumped by a tramcar and caught by the cowcatcher. Dr McIntosh (not then qualified), with a glint in his eye, pushed me forward into the crowd that had gathered, with the words, "This is a doctor!"

I looked at the man. He seemed to be all right and stumped off in the direction of the Grassmarket where, no doubt, he lived in a lodging house. I don't know who he was.

I suppose today the police would have arrived and the paramedics. The tram would have been delayed more than the five minutes!

I expect the tram driver reported the incident to the manager at the end of his shift. He just reset the cowcatcher and went off.

That was my first patient!

It was after Dr McIntosh's departure that Dr Robert A Marshall (below) came to work in Newcastleton in 1960.

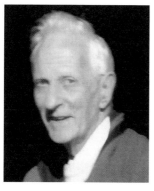

Just at the right time, Dr Murdoch's widow decided to leave Newcastleton and go to Edinburgh.

I was able to purchase Northfield as my mother had died the year before and left me enough money to cover the cost.

(On the occasion of my mother's funeral we were appalled that, with the hearse standing in the front garden of Holmhead, and while Dick Lyth, vicar of Nicholforest conducted a small service in the house, there were people waiting in the waiting room for the morning surgery.)

Dr Marshall bought Northfield from me three years later, when he had decided to remain in Newcastleton as a partner in the practice.

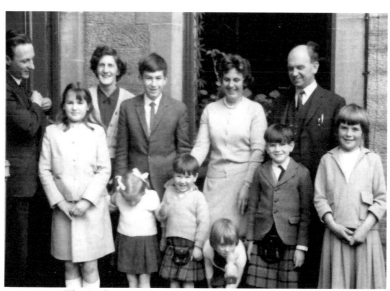

The Bethune and Marshall families, in the early 60s, after Rob had joined the practice as a partner

25. The ambulance service

Back in 1950, the ambulance service was organised quite differently. The ambulance was kept at Cuthberts' Garage (now the Liddesdale garage) and the Cuthberts supplied the driver. This was normally Robbie, but sometimes his father George and later brothers Jim and George when they left the RAF.

Besides responding to emergencies, the ambulance also acted as the hospital car service. The runs were almost all to the Cumberland Infirmary in Carlisle or the Haig Maternity Hospital in Hawick.

The first ambulance was like a large estate car, but later we got a conventional ambulance. If an ambulance was needed, we contacted the Cuthberts directly. Later, double manning arrived and Robbie was joined by George Ferguson, Ian Paterson and Gordon Steele. Ultimately, control was taken over by Dumfries and the ambulance moved to Langholm.

The doctor and the ambulance attended most of the local road accidents, getting there much faster than an ambulance from Langholm or Hawick as is the case today.

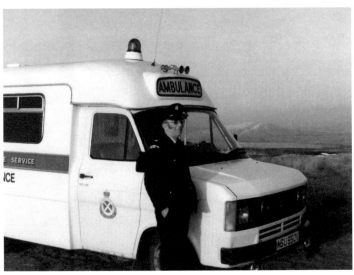

Robbie Cuthbert and the Newcastleton ambulance on the Langholm road, 1983

On one occasion, we had to call out the local fire brigade; a lady with serious injuries had to be cut out of her car. I am glad to say she made an excellent recovery.

Soon after seat belts were introduced, I was

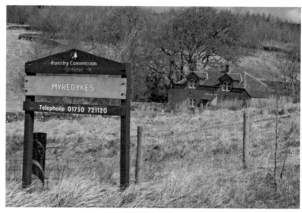

Myredykes, on the road to Kielder

very impressed when a car fell headfirst into the Whitrope Burn, just south of the railway bridge, and the driver was relatively unhurt.

The ambulance carried our pathological specimens to the Infirmary lab. If Robbie was doing a routine run to Carlisle, he came to the surgery to see if there were any specimens to go. In the postal strike of 1971, I made unconventional use of the ambulance - I wrote letters to my sister who worked in the Newcastle hospitals. Robbie gave them to my friend, the transport manager at the Infirmary, who in turn gave them to an ambulance driver going to Newcastle!

It was a sad day when the ambulance service made 'progress' and took away our local ambulance.

Kielder was serviced by the Bellingham ambulance, with Tommy Slee and his wife at Kielder Station providing a hospital car service to take patients to hospital in Hexham, Corbridge or Newcastle.

One Saturday, the Bellingham ambulance could not get to Kielder on account of flooding. This was before Kielder Dam was built. So Robbie and I set off for Kielder with the ambulance.

The road was very badly flooded near Myredykes and we arranged that Andrew Douglas of Saughtree Farm would tow us up to the old railway line at the Caddron Burn. When we got to the spot, Andrew was there with his tractor. "I think you'll get through", he said, and piloted us through the floods.

Twice I have had to come back from Kielder along the railway line because of flooding. Once I drove right across the viaduct (now sadly gone) to Saughtree Station, and the other time just to the Caddron Burn. Dr Marshall also came back by 'rail' once. He had to cut a fence wire across the track!

I also had flooding problems coming back from Roadhead after a flash thunderstorm. I had to turn back at the Knowe Manse and then again up the Bailey near Hillhead, finally getting home via Stonegarthside, to find it had been sunny and dry all day in Newcastleton!

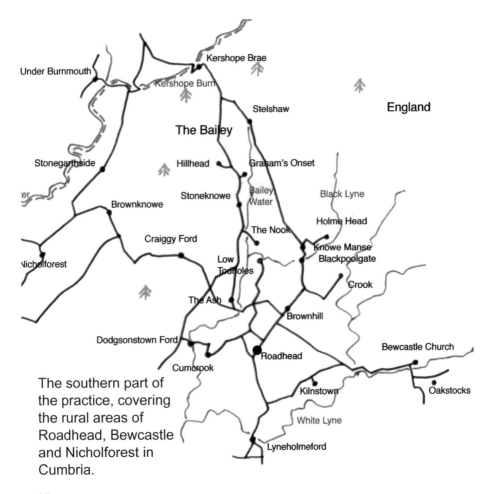

The southern part of the practice, covering the rural areas of Roadhead, Bewcastle and Nicholforest in Cumbria.

26. The practice base

One of the problems of rural general practice before NHS 24, was the manning of the telephone 24 hours a day, seven days a week. In the old days, this was often overcome by having a domestic servant who lived in. This was the case with Dr Evans and Dr Murdoch.

During the working week, we had a full-time employee who worked in the house and also answered the telephone. At other times, reception was shared by my family, or by Zena Weir and the families of other married doctors. We had a telephone exchange in 34 North Hermitage Street with extensions to Fairview and to the doctor's house at 2 Oliver Place.

Later, when Dr Marshall moved into Northfield and the surgery was at Holmhead, we had a very sophisticated phone system (a "Home Exchange") connecting the two houses. I had a big fight with BT to get this facility.

Doris Rutherford was our first employee, followed by Veronica Elliot and finally Jean Davidson. About 1970, the NHS began to give us a grant towards the employment of a receptionist.

Our first full time receptionist was "Punchie", May Cruickshank, whom many likened to Janet of "Dr Finlay's Casebook". Sadly, she died shortly before she was due to retire. She was followed by Bertha Inglis, who continued on at the 4 South Liddel Street surgery after my retirement. An elderly lady, Mrs McGlasson, sometimes kept house for us if we had a locum.

With the surgery attached to our home, Joyce was usually around, and with her nursing and midwifery experience, could tackle emergencies without panicking. For example, Robbie Cuthbert appeared with the ambulance one day en route for Haig Hospital with a patient on the point of giving birth, and she was able to deal with the situation. Joyce controlled the severe bleeding of an elderly lady who had cut her leg badly while splitting logs.

Her greatest triumph was when the butcher appeared minus the tip of his finger. She sent for the fingertip, which was found on the floor of the shop, strapped it back on and it survived!

We had a succession of surgery cleaners, among them Jenny Harkness, Gracie Davidson, Cathie Ireland and, finally, Cecilia Davidson, who continued cleaning right on to the Moss Road days, retiring only last year.

In the early days, both medicine and tablets went out in glass bottles. The bottles were re-cycled and washed (including the corks before the bottles were screw topped). Tablets had to be counted out by hand and we used a plastic counter based on the mathematics of an equilateral triangle. Frances, my daughter, recalls helping to count tablets while she was still a schoolgirl!

I carried quite a lot of tablets on my rounds and would dump some tablets on the table beside a patient's bed and say, for example, "take four a day!"

Medicines dispensed at the surgery went out on the shelf inside the door for patients to collect. One patient, who came every second Wednesday afternoon, started to steal medicines. We knew who she was and we found the missing packets, actually ointments, unopened in her house after she died.

As I have mentioned previously, the drugs came by rail, but delivery became slower and slower, so T&H Smith started to send them by van. Tom, the driver, was a pleasant man but sometimes he would stand for ages telling us how he hadn't enough time. Actually he did have a big round, travelling as far away as Gatehouse-of-Fleet. Later still, the drugs came from the Carlisle depot but were packed in Gateshead!

In the early days, making a phone call to Carlisle meant going through the Langholm exchange, usually manned by a lady called Isa. To phone Roadhead, you went through Carlisle and Langholm, and for Kielder it was Carlisle, Langhom and Hexham!

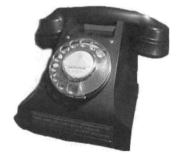

There was a man in the Carlisle exchange who always wanted to know what was going on in Copshaw.

Sometimes while waiting for your call to be put through, you could overhear other conversations. Once I heard a well-known local man describing what the doctor had said. It was remarkably different from what I had actually said!

The arrival of an "ansafone" was a great advance. It meant the doctor could be on call without back-up. The system allowed us to phone in from the country and collect any messages. At one time we tried pagers, but there were too many 'black holes' for them to be useful.

27. Animals

"Please look in on your way back from Roadhead", was the message I received from Mrs Mackenzie, wife of the gamekeeper at Stelshaw Lodge.

On arrival I found the patient was her old Border Terrier! He was very ill. I listened to his chest. Both lungs were solid with pneumonia. I'm afraid he died a few hours later.

With so much contact with the farming community, I was often asked for advice.

Jimmie Waugh of Kilnstown took me out into a field to see a breathless young bull. I didn't know what was wrong, but the Vet later diagnosed tonsillitis.

Stelshaw Lodge

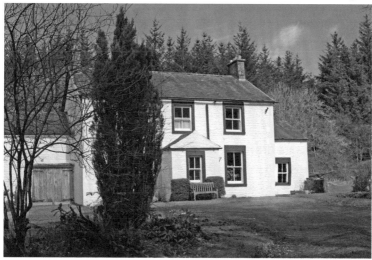

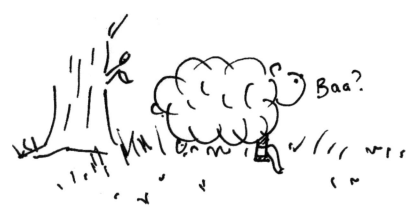

Baa?

At the out-bye Peel Farm, I helped to splint a sheep's broken leg.

Dave Ewart, retired shepherd, used to keep Holmhead garden free of moles, and I was able, in return, to cure his collie's skin irritation.

One morning, I diagnosed that my own West Highland Terrier (Katie, right) had a strangulated hernia and Ken McNaughton, the Longtown vet, did a wonderful job of saving her life, although she had several inches of devitalised intestine.

Twice, I have been asked to put dogs to sleep!

One day I was examining a patient in bed. There was a noise under the bed and an Alsatian emerged. However, it took one look at me and rushed out of the room and straight up

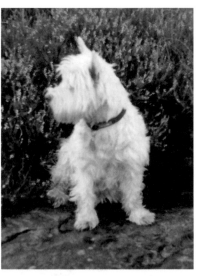

the stairs. I didn't have any problems with Alsatians. I stood on one's paw once and it ran off howling. I was even able to hold one of Daphne Kyle's fierce Alsatians by the collar! I found that small dogs were more aggressive.

The only animals I am really scared of are horses.

The last "medical" work I did after my retirement, was to stitch up a cut on a dog which had been attacked by a larger dog, in the South Liddel Street surgery.

On the way to The Peel farm there was a hundred yards of field to cross. Imagine my consternation when I observed a bull in the field. There was no way round, so I set off, but soon realised the bull was in the next field; the dividing fence was obscured by being in a ditch!

It reminded me of Pilgrim in John Bunyan's "Pilgrim's Progress" when he observed two lions in the way, but found them chained when he reached them.

Under certain weather conditions, I had to walk to Sundhope Farm. On the way, a couple of hundred yards of field had to be crossed and three geese used to come hissing at me.

Brownknowe farmhouse in Nicholforest stood about 15 yards back from the road. That space was patrolled by three greyhounds.

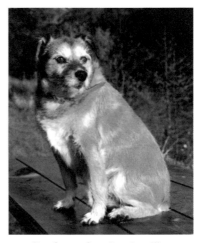

Sandy, my last "patient!"

(Many farms reared them at that time). Greyhounds are friendly and the three used to jump up on me with their muddy paws. The medical bag was useful to keep them at bay!

Coming out of Stoneknowe farm one day, I found seven turkeys perched on the car. I managed to chase away the three on the bonnet, but the four on the roof stayed on until I drove off!

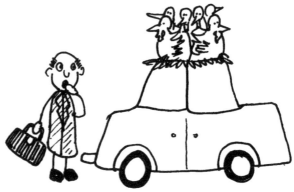

Katie, the best of our Westies, the one who had the hernia, used to get upset if she heard children crying in the surgery. On one such occasion she managed to get through and appeared in the consulting room. The crying child saw her and the tears stopped.

Another way to soothe difficult children was to fill the ear syringe up with water, open the window, and squirt the stream of water high into the garden. Very effective it was! It also amused the doctor! He obviously hadn't grown up.

One of my patients, who kept goats, extolled to me the value of goat's milk in the treatment of eczema and asthma. When he appeared in the surgery one day suffering from eczema, I could not resist the temptation to ask if he had not tried goat's milk. He laughed and enjoyed the joke. There is a place for humour in medicine, but you have to know your patients well, and to know when it is not appropriate.

Some will remember "The Yank", the Penton roadman. (Sadly, he died in a motorbike accident). He sent for me one day. On arrival, he said, "I didn't really need you. I can have three days off sick without a doctor's certificate, but I need your help to fill the form." It was so ludicrous, I could only laugh.

Giving an old lady a liver injection one day, there was a strange sound behind the door. Her daughter flung open the door and found the granddaughter and her friend trying to peer through the keyhole to see what was happening. Now a senior citizen, I expect that friend recalls being caught!

28. Away from the surgery

The work of a GP takes you into the "big house" and also into the lowliest "but and ben". You see people as they really are, especially in emergencies.

I have already mentioned being in a gypsy caravan.

I have also crawled into a tinker's low tent to see a sick child.

I have examined a man's chest in the middle of a hayfield in North Uist, and also been called to accidents in the forest.

The doctor's old-fashioned bag comes into its own then. You can put it down on the ground in the middle of a road, the middle of a field, the middle of a forest, as well as on a patient's bed. (Although twice I have had it kicked off onto the floor with some spillage of the contents.)

I drove a Singer Chamois (see p.80) for some time. There was a level area over the rear engine. One day I came out of a house at Roadhead, placed my bag on this area while I unlocked the car – then drove off! The bag fell off 100 yards up the road but I didn't miss it until I got to Holmehead (Roadhead), two miles away!

Off duty, you are not immune. I have been called out of a sleeper berth on the train to Inverness to see a man who was having a fit. I also dealt with an emergency in the SMT garage at Carlisle. This resulted in my receiving "red carpet" treatment on subsequent visits.

On a Donegal caravan site, I was asked to see a neighbour's child with suspected appendicitis.

Duties also took us into the police station, sometimes to examine someone who had been arrested and who claimed to be ill, sometimes to decide if a suspect was incapable of driving a car due to alcohol. We were very relieved when blood testing came in and all we had to do was to take blood off and not express an opinion.

We had regular patients from Taylor's Shows on their annual week in the park at the Holm Show time. They had five practices where they attended on their annual circuit. We were one. Dr Quarmby of Ambleside was another. The patriarchs of the shows were Billy, brother Matty and sister Dolly. Billy was the boss. He was often ill and once kept the Shows here for an extra week so that I could attend him.

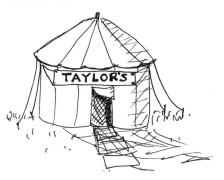

Billy's caravan was an old wooden one with a safe bolted to the floor and bags of coin on the dressers. I often sat in the caravan and learned about show business. Matty was the last to die, and the Shows stopped coming after that.

When I first came to Newcastleton, petrol was rationed and few people had motor cars, so we had to go to people at home. Correspondingly, surgeries were much smaller.

Quite a lot of cottages were off the road and had only a path or track (unsuitable for motors) leading to them. Many were about 100 yards off the road; six were half a mile, and three (or four in snow) about a mile. Black Lyne was two miles walk from Stelshaw Lodge - there was no forestry road then; you just followed the forestry telephone line.

Fortunately, the Waughs decided to move to a herding in the Wythop valley near Bassenthwaite in the Lake District. I have actually walked over that area (Sale Fell) once.

The walk of half a mile from Whitrope Tunnel to Windshielknowe was the most exposed and I have sheltered behind a dyke when a storm of driving hail hit me.

We had an unsolved mystery at Windshielknowe when a boy, who had not been away from his home for weeks, developed measles.

Do sheep carry measles?!

Out visiting patients,
Wellington Ford, 1955

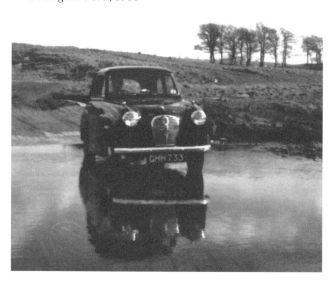

29. *Adventures in the snow*

Out visiting through deep snowdrifts, winter 1961

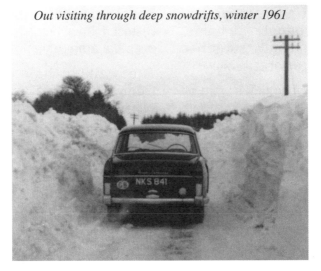

I have already written about flooding, but snow could cause real problems. We seem to have had worse winters in the past than we have now.

One Saturday morning, I had a call to beyond Roadhead. Reaching Blackpoolgate, I found the 100 yards of road beyond were solid with snow. Bill Broatch, the roadman, and Bob Davidson and Douglas Weir in the butcher's van, were there, and the four of us handcut the 100 yards up the hill.

Half a mile further on, I ran into a deep drift outside Brownhill Cottage and had to dig myself out of it. That dear old Christian, Lizzie Armstrong, who lived there, shouted me in as she had a boiled egg and toast ready for me.

It had taken about five hours to make that call to Lyneholmford.

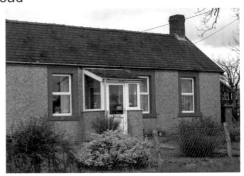

Brownhill Cottage

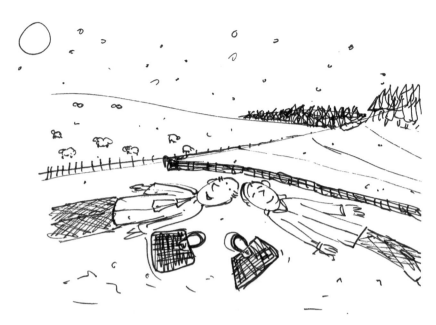

One snowy night, Dr Marshall and I set off for Plashetts (now under the Kielder reservoir). I was driving and when I turned into the Plashetts road, the car said "enough" and spun round to face home. We got out to walk the remaining half mile.

At the top of the hill, I said, "Is it slippy on your side of the road?"

Rob said, "No", and promptly landed on his back.

As I started to laugh, my own foot slipped and there we were, one on each side of the road, laughing our heads off in the moonlight. (The snow had stopped).

Our little patient had pneumonia so it was well worth all the effort.

Another snowy night I was guided over the hill to Redmoss by one of the young Thomson men from Gillside. The snow was so deep that we walked right over the top of a stone dyke on the way.

Coming up from Bewcastle one day, I found the road blocked by the school minibus stuck in the snow. This was at Heather House, and I spent a couple of hours with the children who were having fun playing games in the farmhouse kitchen.

Essential kit for travelling in the snow is a spade or shovel, some sacking or old carpet to put under your wheels to grip on the road when stuck, and a fertiliser bag.

It was old Mr Dobson who introduced me to this after I had walked the mile over the fields from Roadhead to Cumcrook (below) as the loaning was completely blown in.

I had crossed some fences with difficulty but a fertiliser bag enables you to cross barbed wired and electric fences easily.

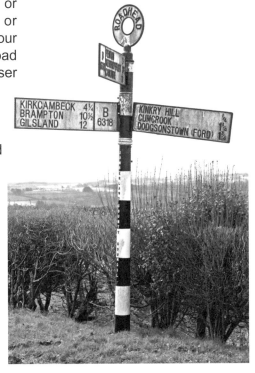

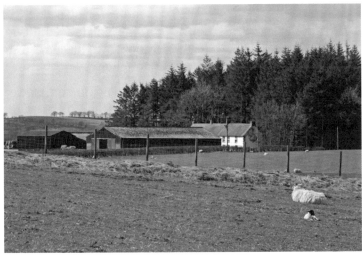

Cumcrook on a bright Spring day, with no snow in sight!

In the days when the Forestry Commission was controlled locally, they were very helpful. One snowy night, they sent a Land Rover to Saughtree to convey Dr Marshall to East Kielder, a shepherd's cottage 1½ miles up in the forest above Kielder Castle.

On another occasion, a Forestry squad took me in the snow to Riccarton Junction and took the patient (the last inhabitant at Riccarton) out to the Limekiln Edge to meet the ambulance.

One call to Low Todholes took four hours to complete. This time it was black ice on the road. My sister, May, was with me, and on the way home we got stuck at Stelshaw farm. We couldn't get away so we turned back and went round by Stonegarthside, but got stuck again, this time on the Pin Brae at the Kershope Burn.

After I had reversed gingerly down, "Jiggs" Thomson (Billy the grocer) came along. "I can get up", he said, but he did not get as far as I had. Billy put his foot on the accelerator and reversed down full speed on the ice. How he stayed on the road was a miracle. Dorothy, his wife, shut her eyes!

So we set off to go home by Burnmouth, with Billy leading. He came over the brow of the hill at Kershopefoot fast. The crossing gates were shut, but the signal man had the presence of mind to swiftly open the gates and Billy shot through!

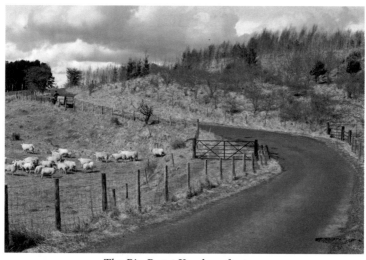

The Pin Brae, Kershopefoot

Kershope Brae was a problem. The Holm squad kept the roads well but it was galling to reach Kershope Burn and find the steep hill on the English side unploughed. Twice I have stuck at the last bend and had

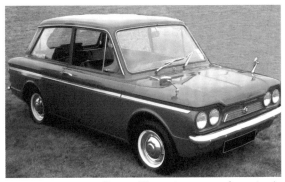

a Singer Chamois - snow champion!

to reverse the whole way down with my hair standing on end!

Tubeless and winter tyres were a great advantage for snow travel. My best car in snow was the Singer Chamois (a de luxe Hillman Imp) on which I put chunky SP44 tyres all round for the winter. On the negative side, cars have less clearance now. With the old Austins, you could bash through almost a foot of snow.

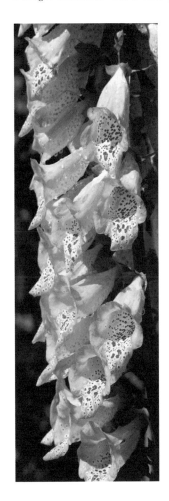

But the snow goes and most days it was a delight to travel round the countryside; watching the lambs grow in the fields, looking for the little banks where violets came up each year, for the yellow marsh marigolds appearing in the ditches, the pimpernels at the Dodgsontown ford, foxgloves at the edge of the forest and there was the smell of the garlic plants on the Hawick road.

30. School contacts
(and an operation on a kitchen table)

It was an ordinary village kitchen. The kitchen is gone, its site occupied by an extension of the neighbouring shop.

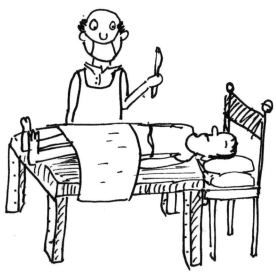

"Mr Maclean," said the 92-year-old man lying on the kitchen table, "I fear going to Carlisle more than your knife."

Mr Maclean was a surgeon from the Cumberland Infirmary who was about to operate and repair the man's hernia with local anaesthesia. The operation was successful.

The elderly lady who looked after the old man told me that, when she was a young lassie at Whithaugh, she disliked school and feigned a headache when it was time to go. But her wise mother said, "Senna tea, then". This was an infusion made by pouring hot water on senna leaves. It was a laxative and had a horrible taste. Her headache disappeared immediately.

Nowadays, we use senna granules that taste better. Table top surgery is a thing of the past, but children still like to skive from school!

One major change occurred in the nursing service after that dearly loved Bewcastle district nurse, Nurse Sanderson, died prematurely. We suggested that instead of having a Longtown-based nurse attend our patients in Bewcastle and Nicholforest, nurses from Newcastleton could attend both.

After a conference with the chief nursing officers from St

Boswells and Carlisle, this was agreed, and the nurses became largely (but not completely) practice based. The chief nursing officer from Carlisle said to me, "You don't realise what you are doing. It has never been known for a district nurse to cross a local authority border, far less a national one!"

The system has worked well. The only problem that arose was the supply of incontinence pads! In Scotland they could be prescribed, but in England they were supplied by the local authority. We were told, "The nurse will have to come to Longtown (15 miles away) to get pads for Cumbrian patients!" We sorted this one out by supplying the pads and charging Cumbria at trade price, but even this simple solution ran into difficulties with the Finance Department at first.

In my early days here, Mr Robin I. Stirling, one of the top Edinburgh Orthopaedic surgeons, whose lectures I had attended as a student, held a children's orthopaedic clinic at the Unionist Club (as the Buccleuch Centre was called). A physiotherapist, whom the children called the "foot nurse", checked the children's feet and their walking at the school, and referred them to the clinic. Some children pretended to walk funnily to get to the clinic. The clinic ceased soon after Mr Stirling's retirement when Mr M. Biagi, surgeon at Peel, took over.

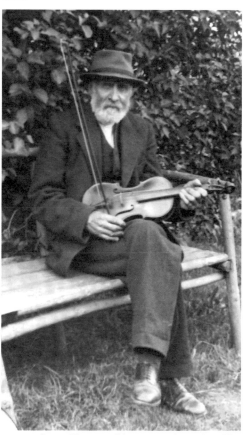

one of two 90 year old patients from the '50s

As doctors, we had quite a lot of contact with the local school. For a while, I was chairman of the Local Education Sub-Committee. Of the headmasters, Bert Petrie introduced me to the new ways of teaching maths, and I was always impressed by the patience Bill Forbes had in handling children with learning difficulties.

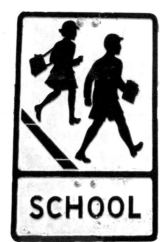

One day, Lorrie Adamson, the school janitor, brought a girl to the surgery. She had pushed a metal key ring onto her finger. I had to cut it off with a ring-cutter which had belonged to Margaret Dalgleish's father and given to me by her mother after his death. The metal was so strong that I had to make two cuts as I could not prise it open after the first cut.

There was an incident when the Hawick school bus collided with a car driven by a director of Manchester City FC. He received severe injuries, but the children were unhurt. As the road was completely blocked and there was nowhere to turn the three buses, I took the responsibility of getting all the children to walk back to the village.

I took their bags and they collected them at Holmhead on the way home. Health and Safety would have a fit now!

Measurements showed it was impossible for the two vehicles to pass on the corner. Joyce, then County Councillor, and the RAC, had been pressing the Council to widen the corner for many months but we were told that it was "a big job" etc. etc. The corner was widened within a week!

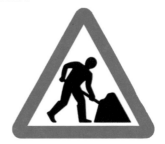

For a while I did the school medical examinations and still draw a pension of 25p per week (increased in 2012 to 75p) for this!

31. Locums

Like everybody else, doctors need holidays, and doctors take ill or have accidents, but patients still need to be cared for.

In the early years of my time here, the two doctors covered each other's absence, but this could be quite exhausting. As the practice grew, however, mainly by the building of many new houses at Kielder, (Castle Drive and Butteryhaugh) we could afford to employ locums. Those houses were filled by young forestry workers from Tyneside, many of whom had young families.

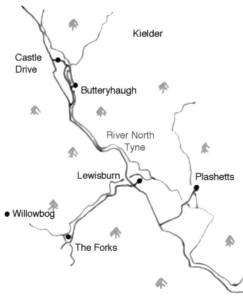

There are (or were) two main sources of locums – adverts in medical journals and agencies like the BMA, or by personal recommendation. Some of the agency recruits were "chronic locums", which often meant they had some personal problem.

One such recruit turned out to be an alcoholic, but despite this he was a very good doctor, though I found him one day at the Dog and Gun on his way to a visit to Kielder. (For readers who do not know the district, the Dog and Gun is five miles in the opposite direction). The last I heard of him was a small piece in the Scotsman stating he had been disqualified from driving for being over the limit!

Another locum had a transverse scar on his head suggesting that he had had a leucotomy, a brain operation in vogue at that time for schizophrenia. He had a mania for "sorting" people's clocks. I am sure many of them never went again!

One day, he asked the mother of a child with impetigo of the face to come to the surgery so that he could apply gentian violet. When another child of similar age arrived, he immediately dabbed his face with the purple dye without making sure it was the correct child!

Another locum, an Indian, was a master at chess and taught my children a lot about the game. He would start the game without his own queen, and still beat you!

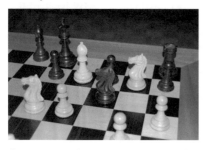

Some good locums came with personal recommendation -

Dr Graham Martin, who became a missionary in Ethiopia before settling down as a GP in Nuneaton;

Dr Kathleen Merricks, who came many times and became a close personal friend;

and Dr Marshall's father, who had been a GP in Dumfries before he retired.

One excellent source of locums

was the Paediatric Dept. of Newcastle where my sister was working. We had many junior doctors from there who would come for spells between hospital appointments. They were all keen. General Practice was new to them and, of course, there was one of us here to guide them. They were able, in return, to tell us about some of the latest developments in medicine.

Some had interesting hobbies. One was a lepidopterist and set up a moth trap in Holmhead garden, just like Mrs Taylor at Riccarton Bar. Later, he worked in different places just to add to his moth collection!

Another young doctor, Leo Kinlen, was very interested in birds and tried to catch dippers. Later, he became head of Epidemiology in Oxford.

Some of these young doctors became consultants in Paediatrics – in Newcastle, Durham and Dumfries.

Others became GPs – Mike McKendrick in Hexham, and Mike Reece in Hartlepool.

Another young locum went on to be a Chest Physician in Edinburgh and, of course, I first came to Newcastleton as a locum!

32. Medicine or Maths?

It is 67 years since I qualified as a doctor at the age of 21, and 72 years since I went to Edinburgh University to study medicine. Because of the wartime necessity to produce more doctors, 20 of us were put on an accelerated course and qualified in four years and four months (instead of the usual five or six years). It was tough going …

I have lived through the most outstanding periods of changes in medicine, some of doubtful benefit, but mostly good, and I have commented on much of this in previous chapters.

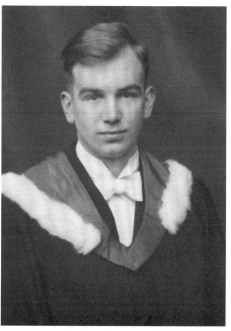

graduation photograph, 1945

One question remains to be answered. Why did this 16-year-old boy who was mad on mathematics, who spent more than half his time in the final years at school doing maths, and who was twice up before George Robertson, the headmaster, for skipping physical education to sit in behind a maths class, suddenly switch to medicine?

My sister, May, was a doctor ahead of me, and she was always encouraging me to do medicine, but the breakthrough came in my visits to Peel Hospital as already described, wandering in the wards (impossible today!)

I came in contact with ill people for the first time, and at the head of each patient's bed was a sheet of "graph paper", better known as a clinical chart. The graphs showed the patient's blood pressure, heart, pulse and respiratory rates and even the number of times they went to the loo!

Here was mathematics - medicine was a branch of mathematics! I would learn at a later date it was a bit more complex than that!

Strangely, my son David made the opposite change. From planning to do medicine, he changed to a 1st class Honours degree in Physics.

Was medicine in the air in my school class at Watsons? Seven of us became doctors – two GPs, four consultants (one a professor of paediatrics) and one the top microbiologist in Scotland.

It was a remarkable class as it also produced three Church of Scotland ministers; Tom Cottrell, the first Principal of Stirling University; Sir Donald McCallum, head of Ferranti's and several lawyers, two of whom became Law Lords.

Then why general practice?

I went to university with the vague idea I would end up as a medical missionary. As a child at Sunday School, I had been entranced by the visit of two missionaries from North India with slides of some remote mountainous areas. In my 'digs' at Lockerbie (my first general practice), I found in the bookcase the life story of Dr Andrew Young, who had lived at Crossdykes near Lockerbie, and had spent his lifetime in China with the Baptist Missionary Society.

I applied to the BMS, but I was in North Uist when the interview was arranged, and made the 39 hour journey (12 in the steamer "Lochmor", and 25 hours in the train) to London for this. I was accepted. I spent the next 18 months doing surgery and midwifery in Dumfries in preparation, but at the end of that time my deteriorating health made going abroad impossible and so I turned to general practice – Creetown, Ibstock (Leicestershire) and finally Newcastleton.

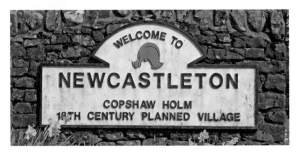

33. A special kind of medicine

General Practice differs from all other branches of medicine in that you may be faced with any type of illness when your patient walks into surgery. The specialist has had his patients sifted out, and some specialists are not so good at general medicine. One very good neurologist for whom I worked at the Western General Hospital asked me to take a patient's blood pressure and to listen to his heart. "I do not know anything about these things!" he said.

The specialist may see a patient once or twice and may never see them again and never know what ultimately happens. The family doctor knows the whole story, what has happened before and after. Does the patient make a full recovery? He may find as the disease progresses that the specialist has made the wrong diagnosis.

60 years ago, one of our patients dropped dead on the way home from hospital. We got a letter the next morning to say that he had no heart trouble!

Don't get me wrong! The specialist is usually correct, and a GP can make mistakes, but the GP has to live with his mistakes!

Pre-NHS 24, as members of a two-man partnership, we were each on call every second night and every second weekend. This limited your social life and that of your family. Only every second weekend were you able to go off somewhere with your family. Perhaps this is why many doctors were keen gardeners. You could garden *and* be on call. Similarly, Joyce and I often played tennis in Holmhead garden when on call.

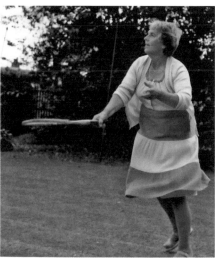

Joyce playing tennis at Holmhead

Lots of teenagers used to play tennis in our garden as well.

You could become very tired, especially if you had been out during the night and then had a full day's work ahead of you – and that day could be long.

During one 'flu epidemic, I remember drinking tea from a flask in the moonlight at 7 pm at Willowbog (3½ miles up a forestry road from Lewisburn) with the prospect of a ¾ hour drive home.

On another occasion after evening surgery, which finished at 7 pm, I had visits at Hillhouse, The Ash (Roadhead) and Kielder.

When I finally reached Kielder about 10.30 pm, the house was in darkness and all had gone to bed – despite their insistence that a call was needed that night, and my informing them I would be very late.

The up side of general practice was that you were there to help people in their time of need. They became your friends. You knew how they lived at home. Were there domestic problems that aggravated their illness? They didn't have to hide the football pools coupon behind the mantelpiece clock as they used to do when the Minister arrived!

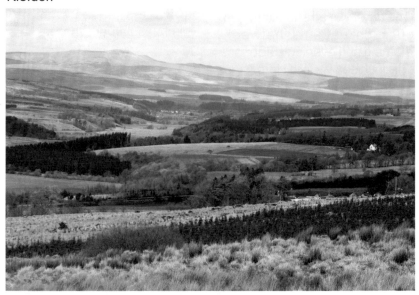

Looking up Liddesdale from Penton at the southern end of the practice. From here to Kielder at the north end of the practice is a drive of over 30 miles.

In my early years here, influenza epidemics were major events. Dozens of people would be ill at once, though the epidemic would be staggered, first appearing in Bewcastle, then in the village, then up Liddel and Hermitage valleys and finally to the very outby cottages. Our aim was to see every case at home. It is foolish to ask people with 'flu to come to the surgery where it could be spread to others. At home, patients would be in bed. It was easy to listen to their chests, examine ears and recognize if they had something else. You could be in and out of the house in five minutes and see a whole family at once.

One day, I visited and examined 50 such patients between morning and evening surgeries. This included visits to Hermitage (four miles to the north) and Grahams Onsett (six miles to the south) - then checked them all again three days later! Most would be well on their way to recovery and you picked out those who had complications.

It amazes me that this exceedingly shy (still is in many ways) little boy (under 2½ stone when he started school at 5½), suffering from repeated childhood illness and never completely fit, could stand up to the stresses and rigours of country general practice. Sidelined at school because I did not worship the god "rugby", I turned to the school Field Club of which I became secretary for two years. We had weekly travel and natural history lectures after school on Thursdays in the winter months, and nature rambles in the summer. We had a nature library and museum.

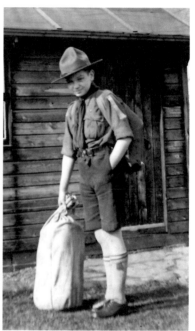

in Scout uniform, 1937

I joined the Cubs and Scouts, became a patrol leader and gained the King's Scout badge.

This all got me out of my shell.

I developed stamina and determination by lots of cycling. (I would have been accepted now in the Chris Hoy era – he went to the same school!) One morning, I cycled the very hilly 49 miles round the Pentland Hills in 4 hours 10 minutes.

Above all, I had my Christian faith and then, what all GPs need - a good wife at home to soothe and encourage when you are tired. I was blessed with a most exceptional one.

Her only fault was to be English!

At the age of 60, I had a series of operations during which I was resuscitated and given four pints of blood. I never regained my full strength and was tired after a busy day, so decided to retire, aged 62, after 40½ years as a doctor.

34. *Did I choose the right career?*

As I approach the end of my reminiscences, the question arises, "Would I choose the same career again?"

Although I entered medicine with a false idea of what it was about, and though I was introduced to general practice by the direction of the Medical War Committee, I cannot imagine doing any other job. It has been a hard life, but a good and fulfilling one. If I was starting now, I am not so sure - there is so much more to learn, and so much more paperwork and bureaucracy, and the ever-present threat of litigation for minor errors of judgement.

If I had pursued a career in maths, and probably obtained an honours degree, what would I have done with it?

Teaching? Spending my life in the classroom? Not for me, although after my retirement, I tutored one young lady for Higher Maths, and enjoyed it immensely. All the thrill of pure maths came back. I even read maths in bed!

More likely, I would have followed my father into the Civil Service, and spent my life as a senior civil servant doctoring statistics for the government!

I had pipe dreams of going back to Uist (I had been asked twice) and, at one time, of doing an Open University degree in maths. But God had a plan for me and for Joyce in Newcastleton, and by a very circuitous pathway we settled here.

My training as a doctor began when I was five. At that age, I was severely mentally traumatised by the action of two doctors, an incident from which it took me 14 years to recover. 84 years later, it's still clear in my mind, even the shape of the windows in the room. I learned that children had to be spoken to and handled gently, and be part of the consultation. I did my best to do that as a doctor. I became suspicious of doctors and learned how to deceive them. At one school medical examination, I stuck my tongue into a huge hole in a tooth and the doctor didn't notice! He was a bit dim or maybe in too much of a hurry. I learned not to let children deceive me. The poacher turned gamekeeper!

One of the fascinations of country general practice is that the unexpected can happen any time. Climbing the Bellevue hill on my way to visit Mrs Mullans of the Bailey Nook (below), I noticed a lot of smoke rising from the farmyard. "Tosh is having a big bonfire", I thought. It *was* a big bonfire - on my arrival I found the hayshed on fire! Tosh and a neighbour had got the cattle away from the yard. I helped get the machinery out but it was unsafe to pull out the blazing hay. When the Fire Brigade arrived they had to run a long hose across the field to the River Black Lyne.

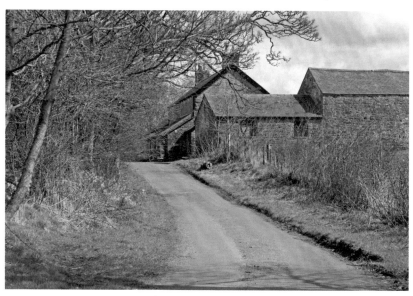

The Bailey Nook Farm

Walking across the moor in North Uist to visit a patient at Locheport, I found a lamb stuck on an island in a small lochan with the ewe lying drowned in the water.

Another surprising thing happened. A lady came to the door in the middle of the night to say her husband was ill and told me exactly what had happened. The surprise was that she had been unable to speak for months after a stroke and afterwards she never spoke again.

I called to see an old lady one evening.

Panic!

She had fallen asleep in her chair and woke up minus her false teeth. She must have swallowed them!

However, an X-ray revealed no teeth inside her. The home help found them in the fire ashes next morning!

Passing a Bewcastle farm one day, I observed a farmer busy at work on the top of a haystack, and I gave him a wave as I passed by.

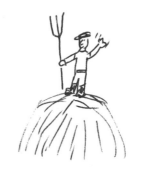

It was four months since his hernia operation and he kept maintaining he was unable to work. I called two days later, did not mention the incident, but he said, "I think I am ready for work now".

(When I was 18, I climbed the seven foot high wall of Dalkeith Palace with the Home Guard, only six weeks after a hernia operation!)

The Secretary of the Communist Party of the state of Victoria in Australia came home to her native Liddesdale, terminally ill. She was a wild restless soul. One day she sat up in bed and said, "Doctor, pray for me." I explained to her the Christian faith. "I can believe that", she said, and for the rest of her illness she was at peace. She said "It's a good job I am going to die, because if I had lived I would have done a great deal of harm."

35. Retirement

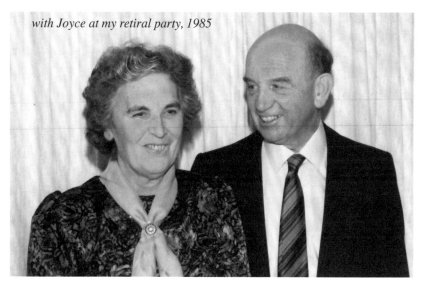

with Joyce at my retiral party, 1985

Yes, general practice was the right career for me, but retirement was even better!

I had time to explore the Liddesdale hills, to take out meals-on-wheels and library books to the housebound.

Joyce and I were able to help at the setting up of Whithaugh Park.

I was chairman of the walks committee of the Heritage Society in its first year and organised the construction of four bridges (built by Dave Lamb), and produced the first walks leaflets.

I was able to give more time to the Congregational Church and other Christian organisations.

Above all, I was able, with the aid of our wonderful Social Works carers, to look after Joyce in her long illness.

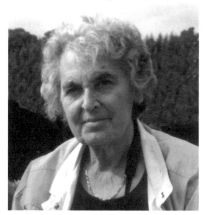

The author

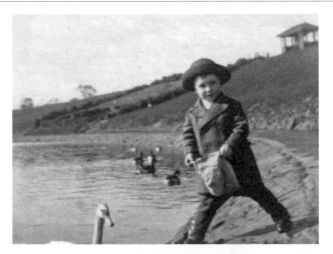

at Inverleith Pond, c. 1927

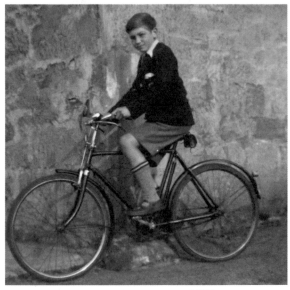

as a teenager, 1937

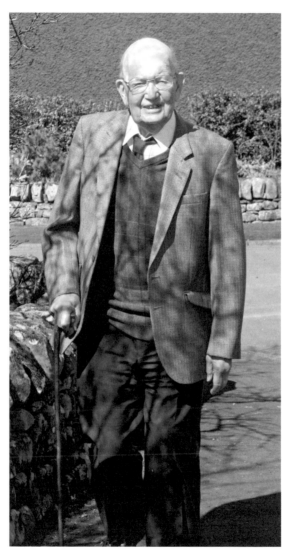

in Newcastleton, 90th birthday, April 2013